HISTOLOGY
Practical Manual

HISTOLOGY
Practical Manual

Sixth Edition

As per the Competency-Based Medical Education Curriculum (NMC)

Balakrishna Shetty MBBS MD
Professor
Department of Anatomy
AJ Institute of Medical Sciences and Research Centre
Mangaluru, Karnataka, India

Sweekritha H Poonja MBBS MD
Associate Professor
Department of Anatomy
AJ Institute of Medical Sciences and Research Centre
Mangaluru, Karnataka, India

Foreword

Chitra Prakash Rao

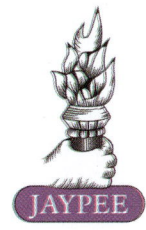

JAYPEE BROTHERS MEDICAL PUBLISHERS

The Health Sciences Publisher

New Delhi | London

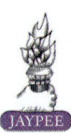
Jaypee Brothers Medical Publishers (P) Ltd

Headquarters
Jaypee Brothers Medical Publishers (P) Ltd
EMCA House
23/23-B, Ansari Road, Daryaganj
New Delhi - 110 002, India
Landline: +91-11-23272143, +91-11-23272703
+91-11-23282021, +91-11-23245672
Email: jaypee@jaypeebrothers.com

Corporate Office
Jaypee Brothers Medical Publishers (P) Ltd
4838/24, Ansari Road, Daryaganj
New Delhi 110 002, India
Phone: +91-11-43574357
Fax: +91-11-43574314
Email: jaypee@jaypeebrothers.com

Overseas Office
J.P. Medical Ltd
83 Victoria Street, London
SW1H 0HW (UK)
Phone: +44 20 3170 8910
Fax: +44 (0)20 3008 6180
Email: info@jpmedpub.com

Website: www.jaypeebrothers.com
Website: www.jaypeedigital.com

© 2024, Jaypee Brothers Medical Publishers

The views and opinions expressed in this book are solely those of the original contributor(s)/author(s) and do not necessarily represent those of editor(s) and publisher of the book.

All rights reserved. No part of this publication may be reproduced, stored or transmitted in any form or by any means, electronic, mechanical, photocopying, recording or otherwise, without the prior permission in writing of the publishers.

All brand names and product names used in this book are trade names, service marks, trademarks or registered trademarks of their respective owners. The publisher is not associated with any product or vendor mentioned in this book.

Medical knowledge and practice change constantly. This book is designed to provide accurate, authoritative information about the subject matter in question. However, readers are advised to check the most current information available on procedures included and check information from the manufacturer of each product to be administered, to verify the recommended dose, formula, method and duration of administration, adverse effects and contraindications. It is the responsibility of the practitioner to take all appropriate safety precautions. Neither the publisher nor the author(s)/editor(s) assume any liability for any injury and/or damage to persons or property arising from or related to use of material in this book.

This book is sold on the understanding that the publisher is not engaged in providing professional medical services. If such advice or services are required, the services of a competent medical professional should be sought.

Every effort has been made where necessary to contact holders of copyright to obtain permission to reproduce copyright material. If any have been inadvertently overlooked, the publisher will be pleased to make the necessary arrangements at the first opportunity.

Inquiries for bulk sales may be solicited at: jaypee@jaypeebrothers.com

Histology—Practical Manual

Third Edition : 2018
Reprint : 2018
Fourth Edition : 2019
Reprint : 2021
Fifth Edition : 2023
Sixth Edition : **2024**

ISBN: 978-93-5696-617-8

Printed at Sanat Printers

FOREWORD

I have great pleasure in writing a foreword to this book *Histology—Practical Manual*.

The authors have hand drawn each diagram carefully and also presented the main features essential for medical and dental undergraduate students.

Most histology textbooks and atlases provide photomicrographs and diagrams which aid in understanding this fundamental science. However, students struggle to draw correct diagrams of histology, and this book in my opinion will surely help them.

My best wishes to the authors.

Chitra Prakash Rao
Ex-Professor
Department of Anatomy
AJ Institute of Medical Sciences and
Research Centre Research Centre
Mangaluru, Karnataka, India

PREFACE

Our main objective is to present complicated histology diagrams in a simple and easy manner. Our students are finding it difficult to replicate diagrams from standard textbooks and atlases. Many diagrams are too complicated with minute details which are not required to be drawn in the record books for an undergraduate student. This book contains hand drawn H and E diagrams of all the slides which are included in the syllabus for undergraduate medical students. In the present edition, we have added many new slides covering the curriculum of various universities in India and updated few of them wherever needed. We tried to make large schematic diagrams which are simple and clear to make it easy for students to replicate in their record books.

We have also given short specific identification points for each slide. Few identification points have also been added which are must know for an undergraduate medical student about the structure and function of the tissues.

In this new edition, we have incorporated tables showing comparison of different histological features of related tissues for quick revision during exams.

We have great pleasure in expressing gratitude to all students and teachers who appreciated and supported our work. We appreciate the valuable feedback, we have received for further improvement. Considering the suggestions, we have added pictures of microscopic photographs of slides in this edition of our book *Histology—Practical Manual*.

We hope that this book will help to make histology record drawings easy for most of the students.

We welcome valuable comments and suggestions which will help us in further improving our book.

We humbly acknowledge the support and guidance of Professor Dr Chitra Prakash Rao and Professor Ajay Udyavar.

I am very grateful to the whole team of M/s Jaypee Brothers Medical Publishers (P) Ltd, New Delhi, India, who helped and guided me, Shri Jitendar P Vij (Group Chairman), Mr Ankit Vij (Managing Director), Mr MS Mani (Group President), Dr Madhu Choudhary (Director–Educational Publishing), Ms Pooja Bhandari [Director–Production (Books and Journals)], Ms Sunita Katla (Executive Assistant to Group Chairman and Publishing Manager), Mr Ajay Kumar Sharma [Deputy General Manager (Books and Journals)], Ms Samina Khan (Executive Assistant to Director–Educational Publishing), Mr Rajesh Sharma (Production Coordinator), Ms Seema Dogra (Cover Visualizer), Neha Verma (Graphic Designer), Mr Vakil Khan (Proofreader), Mr Kulwant Singh (Typesetter), Mr Sumit Kumar (Graphic Designer) and their team members, for all their support to work in this project and make it a success. Without their cooperation, I could not have completed this project.

Balakrishna Shetty
Sweekritha H Poonja

CONTENTS

1. Simple Epithelium — **2–3**
2. Stratified Epithelium — **4–9**
   A. Stratified Squamous (Non-Keratinized)
   B. Stratified Squamous (Keratinized)
   C. Transitional Epithelium
3. Connective Tissue — **10–11**
4. Connective Tissue Fibers — **12–13**
5. Adipose Tissue — **14–15**
6. Hyaline Cartilage — **16–17**
7. Elastic Cartilage — **18–19**
8. White Fibrocartilage — **20–21**
9. Bone—Transverse Section — **22–23**
10. Bone—Longitudinal Section — **24–25**
11. Cancellous Bone — **26–27**
12. Skeletal Muscle — **28–29**
13. Cardiac Muscle — **30–31**
14. Smooth Muscle — **32–33**
15. Peripheral Nerve—Transverse Section — **34–35**
16. Peripheral Myelinated Nerve — **36–37**
17. Optic Nerve—Transverse Section — **38–39**
18. Sympathetic Ganglion — **40–41**
19. Dorsal Root Ganglion/Spinal Ganglion — **42–43**
20. Large Artery/Elastic Artery — **44–45**
21. Medium-sized Artery/Muscular Artery — **46–47**
22. Large Vein — **48–49**
23. Medium-sized Vein — **50–51**
24. Capillaries and Sinusoids — **52–53**
25. Lymph Node — **54–55**
26. Spleen — **56–57**
27. Tonsil — **58–59**
28. Thymus — **60–61**
29. Serous Salivary Gland — **62–63**
30. Mucus Salivary Gland — **64–65**
31. Mixed Salivary Gland — **66–67**
32. Thick Skin — **68–69**
33. Thin Skin — **70–71**
34. Hair — **72–73**
35. Trachea — **74–75**
36. Lung — **76–77**
37. Epiglottis — **78–79**
38. Lip — **80–81**
39. Tongue — **82–85**
    A. Filiform and Fungiform Papillae
    B. Circumvallate Papillae
40. Tooth — **86–87**
41. Esophagus — **88–89**
42. Stomach: Fundus and Body — **90–91**
43. Stomach: Pylorus — **92–93**
44. Duodenum — **94–95**
45. Jejunum — **96–97**
46. Ileum — **98–99**
47. Large Intestine — **100–101**
48. Appendix — **102–103**
49. Liver — **104–105**
50. Gallbladder — **106–107**
51. Pancreas — **108–109**
52. Kidney — **110–111**
53. Ureter — **112–113**
54. Urinary Bladder — **114–115**
55. Prostatic Urethra — **116–117**

56. Testis	**118–119**	
57. Epididymis	**120–121**	
58. Ductus Deferens/Vas Deferens	**122–123**	
59. Prostate	**124–125**	
60. Seminal Vesicle	**126–127**	
61. Ovary	**128–129**	
62. Uterus	**130–133**	
A. Proliferative		
B. Secretory		
63. Fallopian Tube	**134–135**	
64. Mammary Gland	**136–141**	
A. Inactive Stage		
B. In Pregnancy		
C. In Lactation		
65. Umbilical Cord	**142–143**	
66. Placenta	**144–145**	
67. Pituitary Gland	**146–147**	
68. Suprarenal/Adrenal Gland	**148–149**	
69. Thyroid and Parathyroid	**150–151**	
70. Cornea	**152–153**	
71. Corneoscleral Junction	**154–155**	
72. Retina	**156–157**	
73. Eyelid	**158–159**	
74. Organ of Corti	**160–161**	
75. Cerebrum	**162–163**	
76. Cerebellum	**164–165**	
77. Spinal Cord	**166–167**	

COMPETENCY TABLE

Number	The student should be able to	Core (Y/N)	Page Number
AN9.2	Breast: Describe the location, extent, deep relations, structure, age changes, blood supply, lymphatic drainage, microanatomy and applied anatomy of breast.	Y	134–139
AN43.2	Identify, describe and draw the microanatomy of pituitary gland, thyroid, parathyroid gland, tongue, salivary glands, tonsil, epiglottis, cornea, retina.	Y	78, 80, 144, 148
AN43.3	Identify, describe and draw microanatomy of olfactory epithelium, eyelid, lip, sclerocorneal junction, optic nerve, cochlea—organ of corti, pineal gland.	N	78, 150–161
AN52.1	Describe and identify the microanatomical features of gastrointestinal system: Esophagus, fundus of stomach, pylorus of stomach, duodenum, jejunum, ileum, large intestine, appendix, liver, gallbladder, pancreas and suprarenal gland.	Y	86–107, 146
AN52.2	Describe and identify the microanatomical features of: Urinary system: Kidney, ureter and urinary bladder. Male reproductive system: Testis, epididymis, vas deferens, prostate and penis. Female reproductive system: Ovary, uterus, uterine tube, cervix, placenta and umbilical cord.	Y	108–113, 114–125, 126–133, 140–143
AN64.1	Describe and identify the microanatomical features of spinal cord, cerebellum and cerebrum.	Y	154–159
AN65.1	Identify epithelium under the microscope and describe the various types that correlate to its function.	Y	2–9
AN66.1	Describe and identify various types of connective tissue with functional correlation.	Y	10–15
AN67.1	Describe and identify various types of muscle under the microscope.	Y	28–33
AN68.1	Describe and identify multipolar and unipolar neuron, ganglia, peripheral nerve.	Y	34–43
AN69.1	Identify elastic and muscular blood vessels, capillaries under the microscope.	Y	44–53
AN70.1	Identify exocrine gland under the microscope and distinguish between serous, mucous and mixed acini.	Y	62–67
AN70.2	Identify the lymphoid tissue under the microscope and describe microanatomy of lymph node, spleen, thymus, tonsil and correlate the structure with function.	Y	54–61
AN71.1	Identify bone under the microscope; classify various types and describe the structure-function correlation of the same.	Y	22–27
AN71.2	Identify cartilage under the microscope and describe various types and structure- function correlation of the same.	Y	16–21
AN72.1	Identify the skin and its appendages under the microscope and correlate the structure with function.	Y	68–73

COMPARE AND CONTRAST MICROSCOPIC FEATURES

I. MUSCLE FIBRES

	Cardiac muscle	*Skeletal muscle*
Muscle fibre	❖ Short cylindrical ❖ Branched	❖ Long cylindrical ❖ Unbranched
Nucleus	❖ Single, oval ❖ Centrally placed	❖ Multiple, flat ❖ peripherally placed
Intercalated disc	Present	Absent
Cross striations	Not prominent	Prominent
Mitochondria	More	Less
T tubules and sarcoplasmic retinaculum	At Z band form dyads	At AI junctions forming triads
Location	Heart	Muscles of limbs, body wall, tongue etc.

II. ARTERIES

	Large artery or Elastic artery	*Medium sized artery or muscular artery*
Layers	3 layers Tunica intima Tunica media Tunica adventitia present	3 layers Tunica intima Tunica media Tunica adventitia present
Tunica media	❖ Thickest ❖ More elastic fibres ❖ Few smooth muscles	❖ Thickest ❖ Few elastic fibres ❖ More smooth muscles fibres
Internal elastic lamina	Less prominent	More prominent
Vasa vasorum	Present	Present
Example	Aorta	❖ Radial artery ❖ Ulnar artery

III. LARGE ARTERY AND LARGE VEIN

	Large artery	*Large vein*
3 Layers **Tunica intima** **Tunica media** **Tunica adventitia**	Present Thick walled	Present But thin walled
Lumen	Patent	Collapsed
Tunica media	❖ Thickest ❖ More smooth muscle and elastic fibres	❖ Thin ❖ Less smooth muscles and elastic fibres
Tunica adventitia	❖ Relatively thin ❖ Absence of longitudinally arranged smooth muscles	❖ Thickest layer ❖ Longitudinally arranged smooth muscles present
Valves	Absent	Present
Example	Aorta	SVC, IVC

IV. LYMPH NODE AND SPLEEN

	Lymph node	**Spleen**
Capsule, trabeculae	Present	Present
Subcapsular sinus	Present	Absent
Divided into	Outer cortex Inner medulla	White pulp and red pulp
Parenchyma	❖ Cortex has lymphoid follicles containing B lymphocytes with germinal center consisting of rapidly dividing B lymphocytes ❖ Paracortex has T lymphocytes ❖ Medulla-- has lymphocytes arranged as cords separated by sinusoids	❖ White pulp--- periarterial lymphatic sheath of T lymphocytes. ❖ Germinal center/ malpighian bodies have B lymphocytes ❖ Red pulp/ Cords of Billroth-- sinusoids surounded by anastomosing cords of lymphocytes
Function	Filtration of lymph	Filtration of blood—removal of old RBC

V. NERVES

	Peripheral nerve	**Optic nerve (cranial nerve)**
Axons	Bundles of myelinated and non myelinated axons	Bundles of myelinated axons of ganglion cells of retina
Central artery and vein of retina	Absent	Present
Coverings	Endoneurium Perineurium Epineurium	Three meninges- dura mater, arachnoid mater, piamater
Myelination	By schwann cells	By oligodentrocytes
Neurilemma	Present	Absent
Regeneration	Possible	Not possible

VI. GANGLIONS

	Spinal ganglion or dorsal root ganglion	**Sympathetic ganglion**
Capsule	Thick	Thin
Arrangement	Cells in groups between nerve fibre bundles	Scattered in between nerve fibres
Cell body	Pseudounipolar	Multipolar
Cell Size	Large	Small
Nucleus	Central	Eccentric nucleus
Satellite cells	More	Few
Location	Dorsal root of spinal nerves	Sympathetic trunk
Function	Sensory neuron (first order)	Belong to autonomic nervous system (contains post ganglion sympathetic neuron)

VII. SEROUS AND MUCOUS GLANDS

	Serous glands	Mucous glands
Acinus	❖ Small ❖ Narrow lumen	❖ Larger ❖ Large lumen
Cells	❖ Pyramidal ❖ Apical part has zymogen ❖ Granules (eosinophillic staining)	❖ Columnar ❖ Apical parts has mucous droplets (pale staining)
Nucleus	Round basal	Flat basal
Biphasic Staining	present	absent
Ducts	More	Less
Secretion	Watery	Thick mucous

VIII. SKIN

	Thick skin	Thin skin
Layers	Epidermis & dermis	Epidermis & dermis
Epidermis	5 layers	3 layers
Keratin layer	Thick	Thin
Hair follicle	Absent	Present
Sebaceous glands	Absent	Present
Arrector pili muscle	Absent	Present
Sweat glands	More	Less
Distribution	Palms and soles	All over body except palms and soles

IX. BRONCHUS AND BRONCHIOLES

	Bronchus	Bronchioles
Size	Larger	Smaller (≤1mm)
Lining epithelium	Pseudostratified columnar	Simple columnar/cuboidal
Cilia	Present	Absent
Goblet cells	Present	Absent
Plates of hyaline cartilage	Present	Absent
Submucosal Glands	Present	Absent
Smooth muscles	Less	More

X. STOMACH - FUNDUS AND PYLORUS

	Fundus	*Pylorus*
4 Layers	Present	Present
Gastric pits	Shallow (1/3 of thickness of mucosa)	Deep (2/3 of thickness of mucosa)
Gastric glands	❖ Simple straight tubular/ branched ❖ Longer glands	❖ Coiled tubular ❖ Shorter
Cells in glands	❖ Parietal cells ❖ Chief/ zymogen cells ❖ Mucus neck cells ❖ Stem cells ❖ Neuro endocrine cells	❖ Mucous secreting cells ❖ Few parietal cells ❖ No zymogen/ chief cells ❖ Stem cells ❖ Neuro endocrine cells

XI. SMALL INTESTINE AND LARGE INTESTINE

	Small intestine	*Large intestine*
Layers	4 layers	4 layers
Villi	present	absent
Lining epithelia	Simple columnar with microvilli	Simple columnar with microvilli
Goblet cells	Present	More than small intestine
Other features	❖ Brunner's glands in duodenum ❖ Peyer's patch in ileum	Scattered lymphoid follicles in lamina propria
Taenia coli	Absent	Present

XII. PCT AND DCT

	PCT (Proximal convoluted tubule)	*DCT (Distal convoluted tubule)*
Size (cross section)	Larger	Smaller
Lining	❖ Simple columnar with brush border ❖ Cells show Eosinophilic staining	❖ Simple cuboidal ❖ Pale staining cells
Lumen	Narrow	Larger

XIII. URETER AND VAS DEFERENS

	Ureter	*Vas deferens*
3 Layers Mucosa muscular layer adventitia	Present	Present
Lumen	Star shaped in transverse sections	Smaller lumen
Lining	Transitional epithelium	Simple columnar cells
Stereocilia	Absent	Present
Function	Conveys urine from kidney to urinary bladder	Transports spermatozoa from epididymis to ejaculatory duct

HISTOLOGY
Practical Manual

1. SIMPLE EPITHELIUM

Single Layer of Cells Resting on a Basement Membrane

Types—depending on the shape of cells:

a. Simple squamous—single layer of flattened cells with flattened nucleus.
   Example: Endothelium, mesothelium, lining of alveoli of lungs.
b. Simple cuboidal—single layer of polygonal cells with equal breadth and height. Cells appear square shaped and have central round nucleus.
   Example: Follicular cells of thyroid, cells lining the collecting ducts of kidney.
c. Simple columnar—single layer of polygonal cells with height greater than width. Cells appear tall with elongated basal nuclei.
   Example: Mucosal lining of stomach and gallbladder.
d. Pseudostratified epithelium—single layer of cells with different height because of which the epithelium appears stratified (many layered).
   Example: Respiratory epithelium.

1. SIMPLE EPITHELIUM

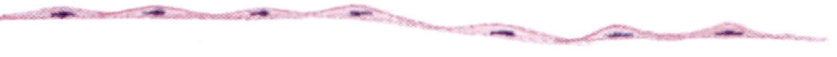
Simple Squamous Epithelium

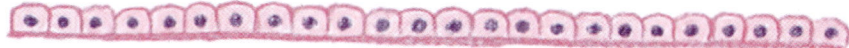
Simple Cuboidal Epithelium

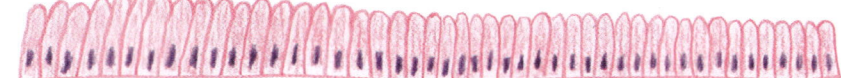
Simple Columnar Epithelium

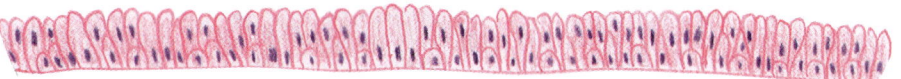
Pseudostratified Columnar Epithelium

2. STRATIFIED EPITHELIUM

2(A): Stratified Squamous
– Non-keratinized

Contains many layers of cells with basal layer resting on a basement membrane

Stratified squamous non-keratinized—contains basal layer of columnar cells, middle layers of polygonal cells and superficial layers of flattened cells.

Example: Mucosal lining of esophagus and oral cavity.

2(A). STRATIFIED SQUAMOUS (NON-KERATINIZED)

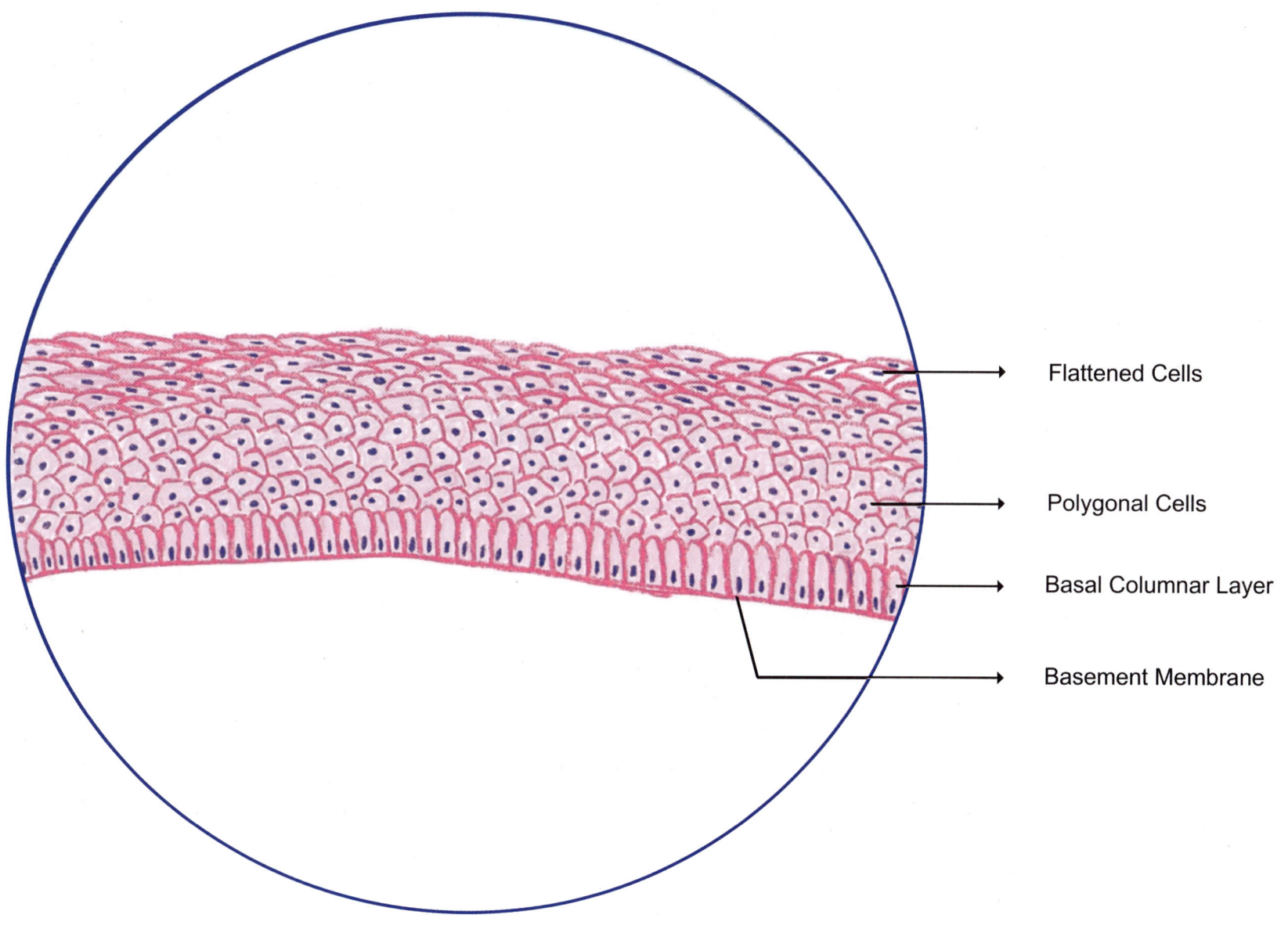

- Flattened Cells
- Polygonal Cells
- Basal Columnar Layer
- Basement Membrane

2. STRATIFIED EPITHELIUM

2(B): Stratified Squamous
– Keratinized

Stratified squamous keratinized—contains basal layer of columnar cells, middle layers of polygonal cells and superficial layers of flattened cells which are keratinized. Topmost layer contains dead cells without nucleus filled with keratin.

Example: Skin.

2(B). STRATIFIED SQUAMOUS (KERATINIZED)

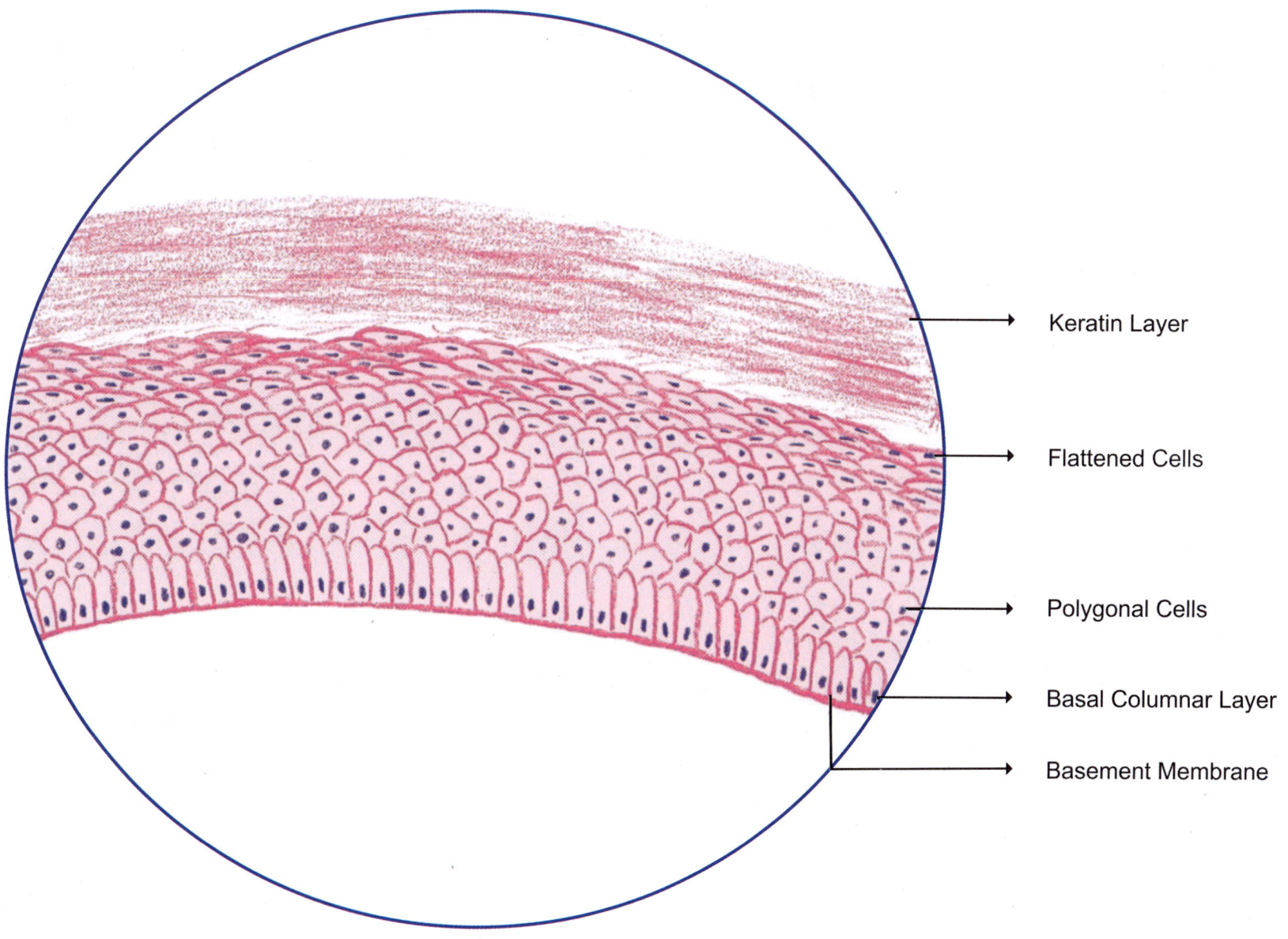

2. STRATIFIED EPITHELIUM

2(C): Transitional Epithelium

Transitional Epithelium
- Five to six layers thick.
- Basal layer of cuboidal cells, middle layers of polygonal cells, superficial layer is made of large dome-shaped or umbrella-shaped cells with single nucleus.
- Unique feature of this epithelium is stretchability and impermeability.

Example: Urothelium—lining of urinary bladder and ureter.

2(C). TRANSITIONAL EPITHELIUM

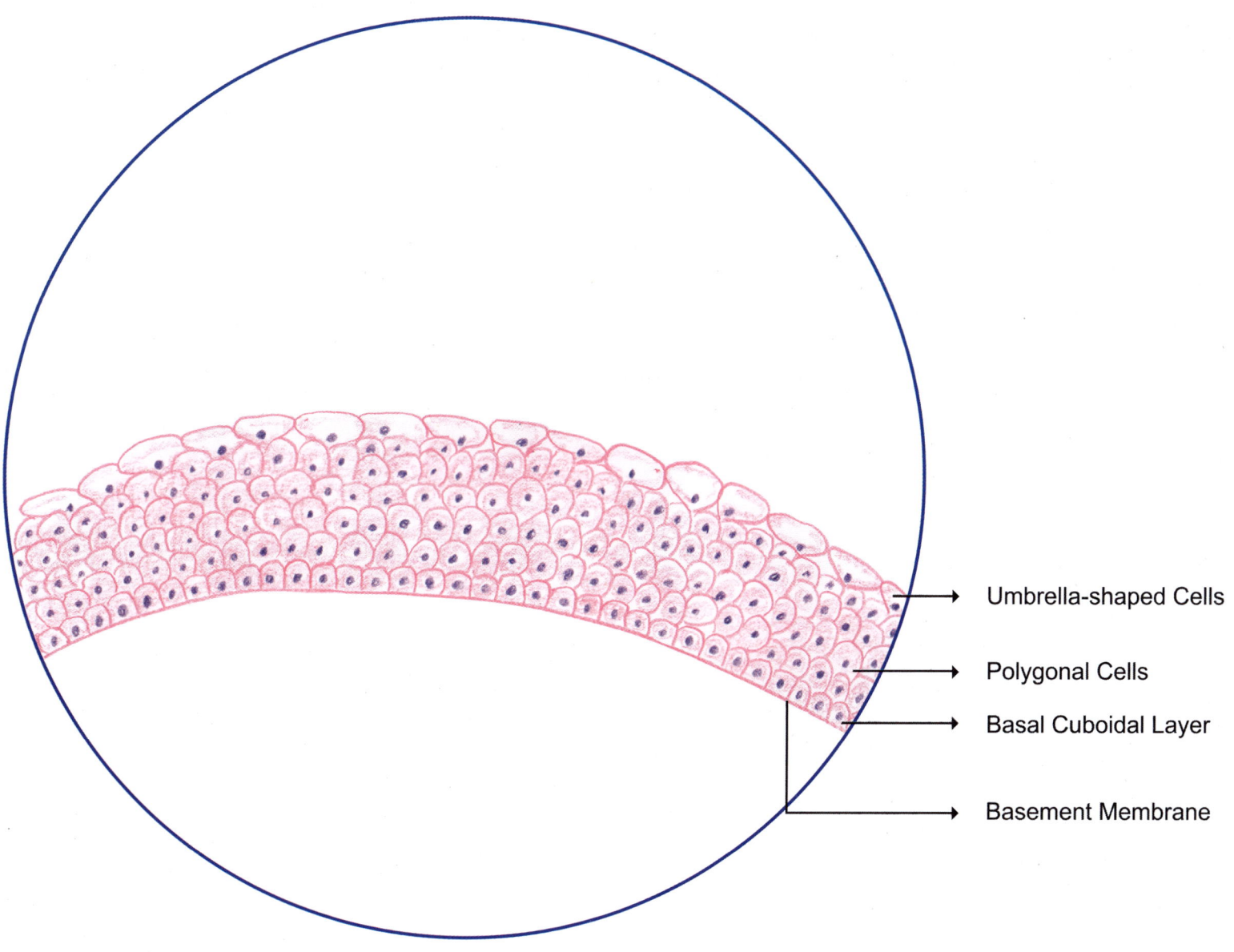

3. CONNECTIVE TISSUE

Connective Tissue

It fills the spaces between the tissues and binds it together. It is made of cells and extracellular matrix. The matrix is made of ground substance and fibers.

1. Cells:
   a. Intrinsic cells—fibroblasts, undifferentiated mesenchymal cells, pigment cells, fat cells.
   b. Extrinsic cells—macrophages, mast cells, lymphocytes, plasma cells, monocytes, eosinophils.
2. Fibers—collagen fibers, elastic fibers and reticular fibers.
3. Ground substance: Viscous material, a complex of carbohydrates and proteins:
   a. Proteogylcans, which is made of gylcosaminoglycans and proteins. Glycosaminoglycans, e.g. chondroitin sulphate, keratan sulphate, hyaluronic acid, dermatan sulphate and heparin sulphate.
   b. Structural proteins—which binds the cells to fibers, e.g. laminin, fibronectin.

- Fibroblasts —are fixed cells, spindle shaped, flat nucleus, show branching processes. Nucleus has prominent nucleoli.
- They synthesise the fibers of connective tissue.

3. CONNECTIVE TISSUE

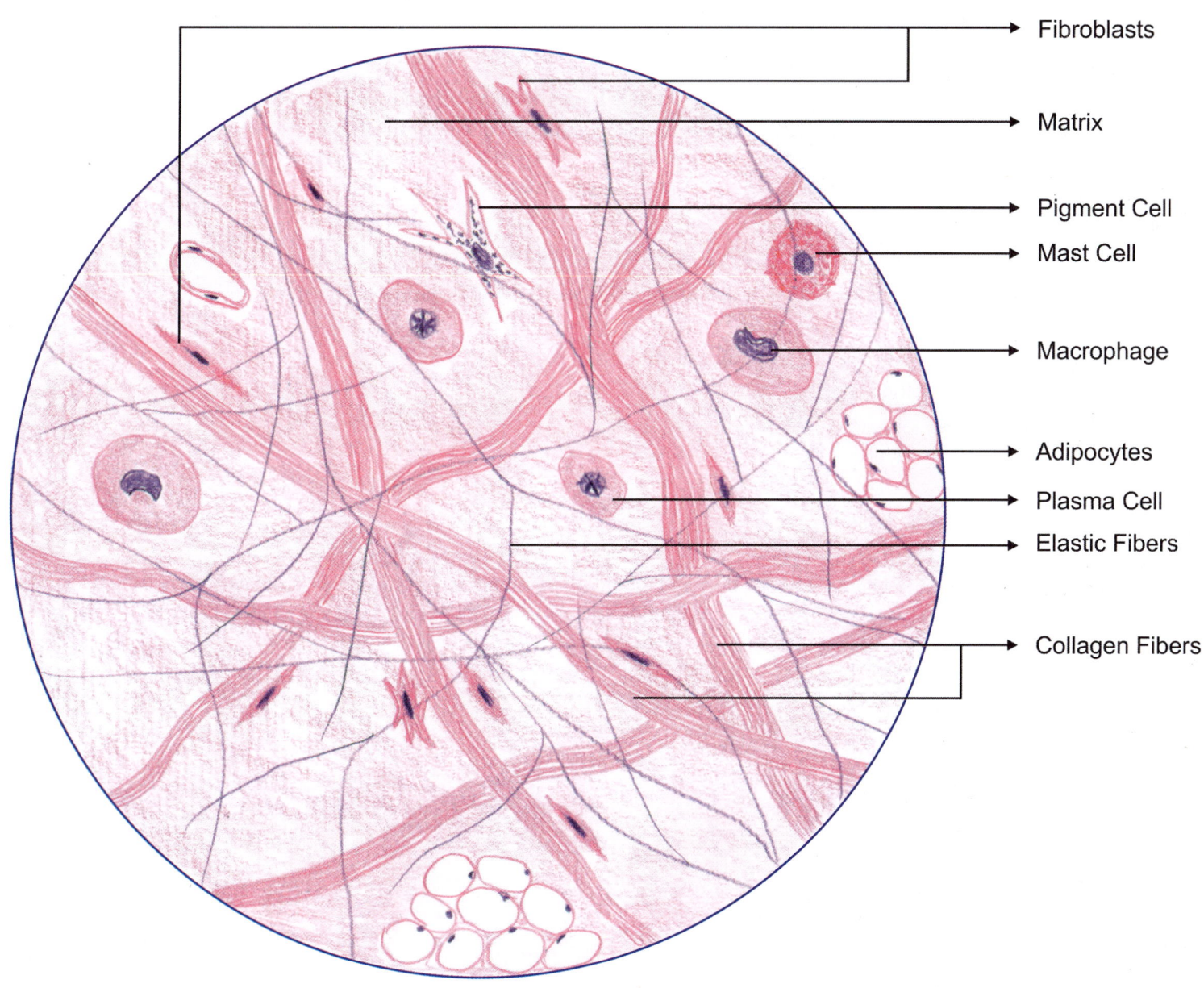

4. CONNECTIVE TISSUE FIBERS

Connective Tissue Fibers

Collagen fibers:
- Most abundant type of fibers. In the form of straight or wavy bundles which branch. But individual fibers do not branch.
- Made up of microfibrils—which contain a collagen protein, further made of smaller subunits called tropocollagen.
- In H&E they stain light pink.
- Produced by fibroblast, chondroblast, osteoblast and smooth muscles of blood vessels.
- Can resist stretching. Found in tendons, bone, ligaments, cartilage.

Elastic fibers:
- They are less than collagen fibers. Run singly and not in bundles. Individual fibers branch and anastomose and form plexus.
- When fibers are cut, the ends retract and recoil.
- Made of protein called elastin which contains smaller subunits of tropoelastin.
- Produced by fibroblast and smooth muscles of blood vessels.
- Ability to stretch and return to original length.
- Found in large arteries, elastic cartilage.

Reticular fibers:
- They are considered as Type III collagen fibers.
- Form a network, branching and anastomosing with each other.
- Found as supporting network in lymphoid organs, glands, kidneys, liver and basement membranes. Produced by fibroblast.

4. CONNECTIVE TISSUE FIBERS

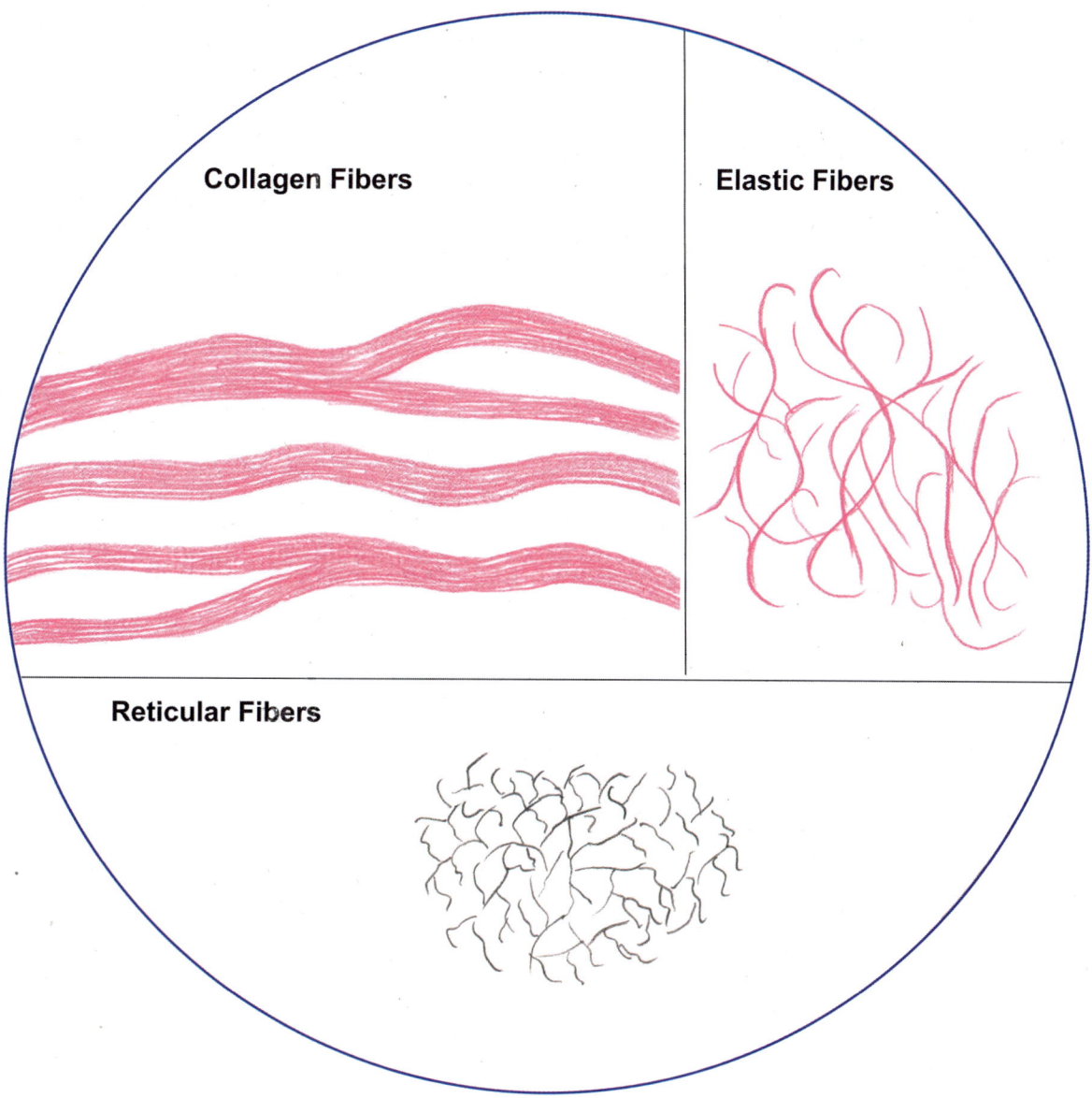

5. ADIPOSE TISSUE

Adipose Tissue

- A group of fat cells is called adipose tissue.
- Fat cells (adipocytes):
  - Specialized for synthesis and storage of fat.
  - Each cell shows a large globule of fat.
  - The nucleus is flattened and pushed to the periphery.
  - The cytoplasm appears as a thin rim around the fat globule giving a signet ring appearance.

5. ADIPOSE TISSUE

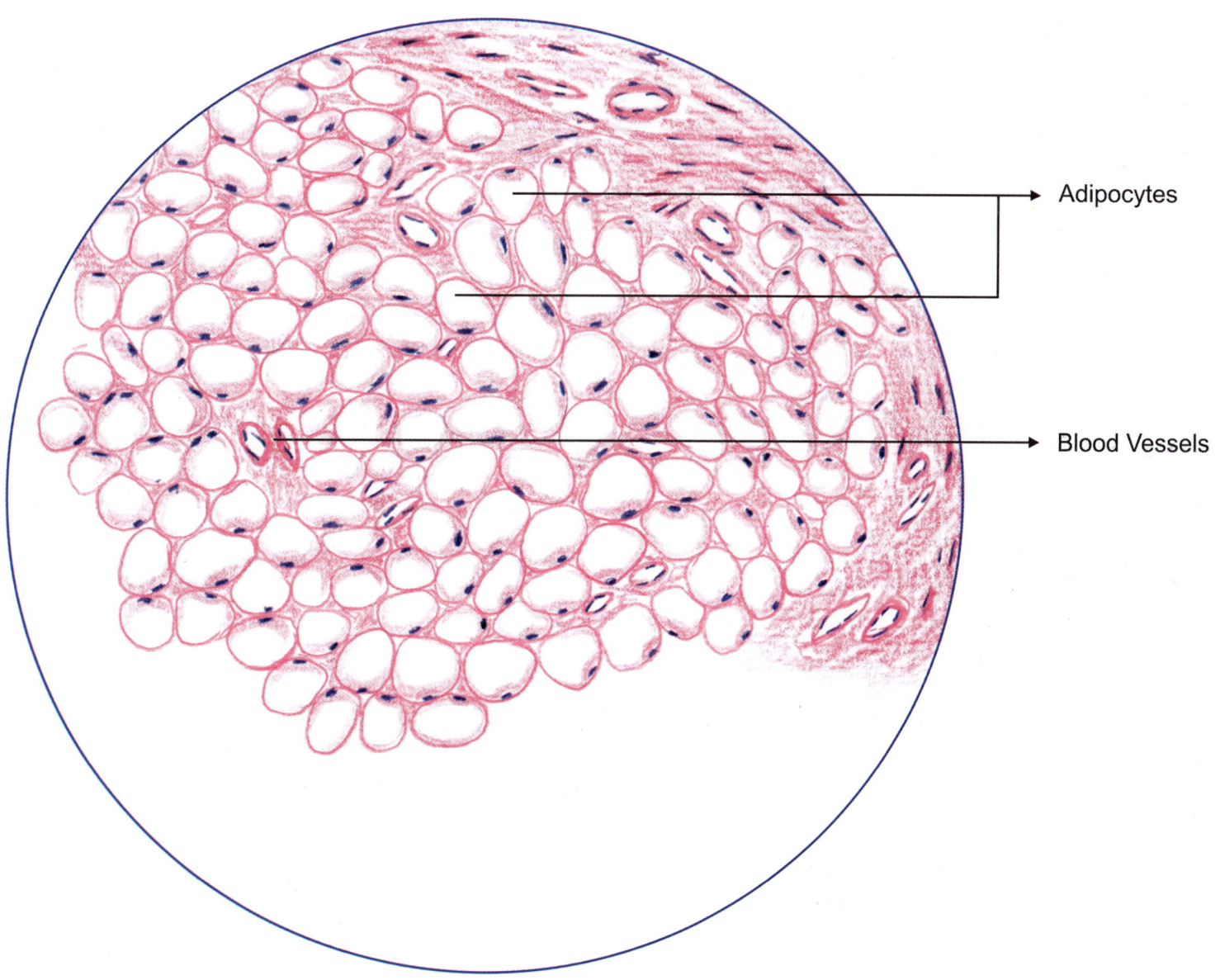

6. HYALINE CARTILAGE

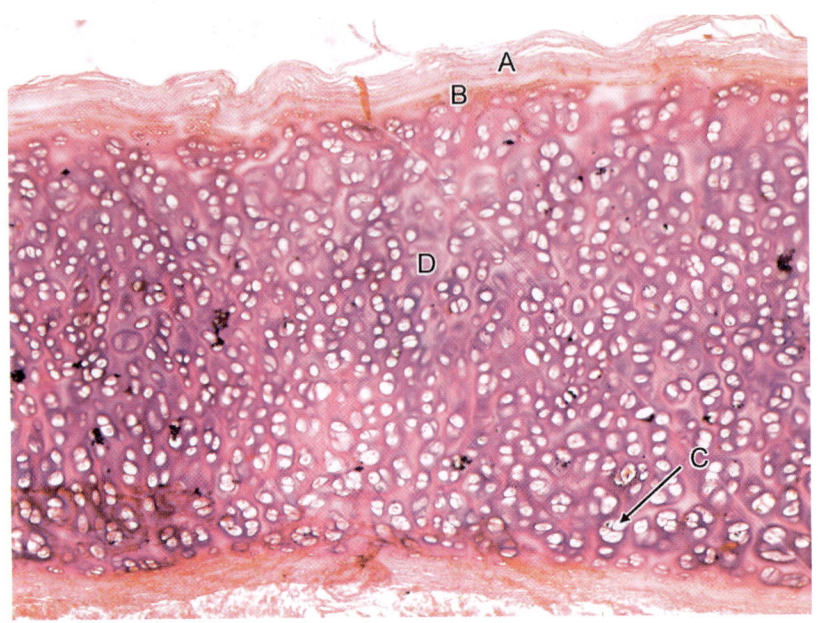

A	Perichondrium—Outer Fibrous Layer
B	Perichondrium—Inner Cellular Layer
C	Chondrocytes in Cell Nests
D	Matrix

Identification Points

1. **Typical chondrocytes in cell nests of 2–4 cells.**
2. **Homogenous basophilic matrix.**
3. **Perichondrium present.**

- Hyaline cartilage has typical ground glass appearance with homogenous bluish matrix.
- Chondrocytes lie within the lacunae. They are arranged in groups of 2–6 cells called cell nest. Apposing surfaces of chondrocytes are flattened.
- Matrix is basophilic due to presence of large amount of proteogylcans and homogenous because the refractive index of collagen fibers and ground substance is same.
- Matrix around the cell nest looks denser and dark staining and is called territorial matrix. It is the newly formed matrix secreted by the chondrocytes.
- In between the nests is the inter-territorial matrix which is pale staining.
- Hyaline cartilage is surrounded by perichondrium which is a two-layered structure—inner cellular and outer fibrous layer.
  - Fibrous layer made of collagen fibers.
  - Cellular layer is made of chondrogenic cells responsible for appositional growth of cartilage.

  Example: Articular cartilage, fetal skeleton, costal cartilage, epiphyseal plate.

6. HYALINE CARTILAGE

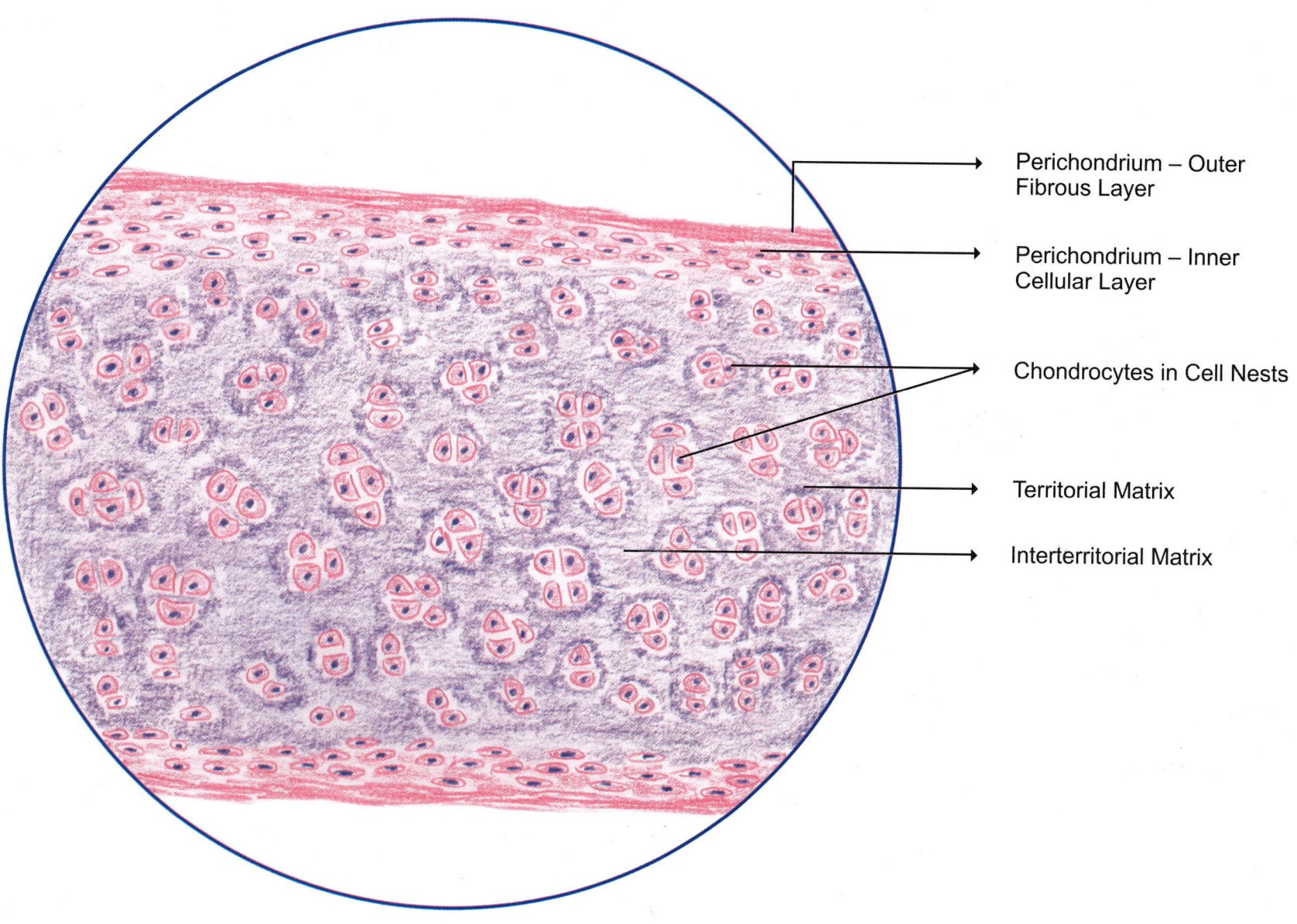

7. ELASTIC CARTILAGE

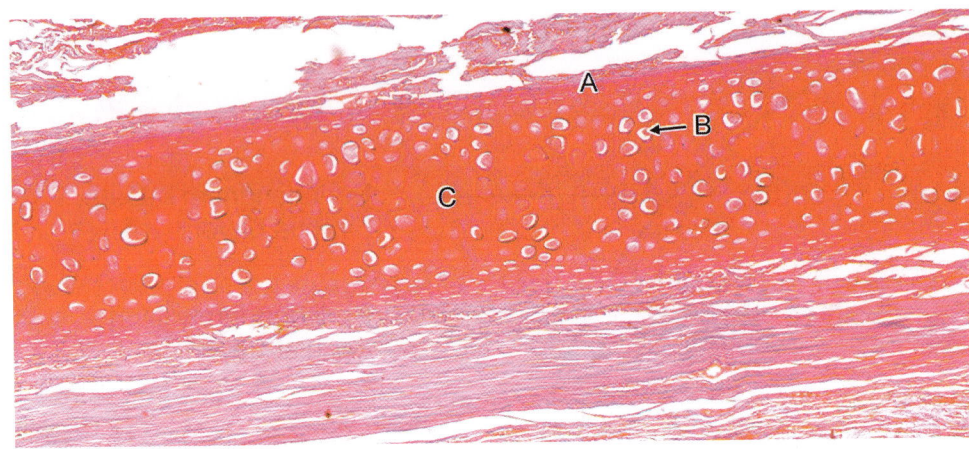

A	Perichondrium—Outer Fibrous Layer
B	Chondrocytes
C	Matrix

Identification Points

1. **Numerous chondrocytes but fewer cell nests.**
2. **Matrix with elastic fibers.**
3. **Perichondrium present.**

- Chondrocytes are large arranged singly or in groups of two within the lacunae. Number of chondrocytes is more in elastic cartilage.
- Matrix in elastic cartilage is eosinophilic with lot of branching elastic fibers.
- Elastic cartilage is surrounded by perichondrium which is a two-layered structure—inner cellular and outer fibrous layer.
  – Fibrous layer made of collagen fibers.
  – Cellular layer is made of chondrogenic cells responsible for appositional growth of cartilage.

Example: Epiglottis, Eustachian tube, external acoustic meatus, external ear, corniculate and cuneiform cartilages of larynx.

7. ELASTIC CARTILAGE

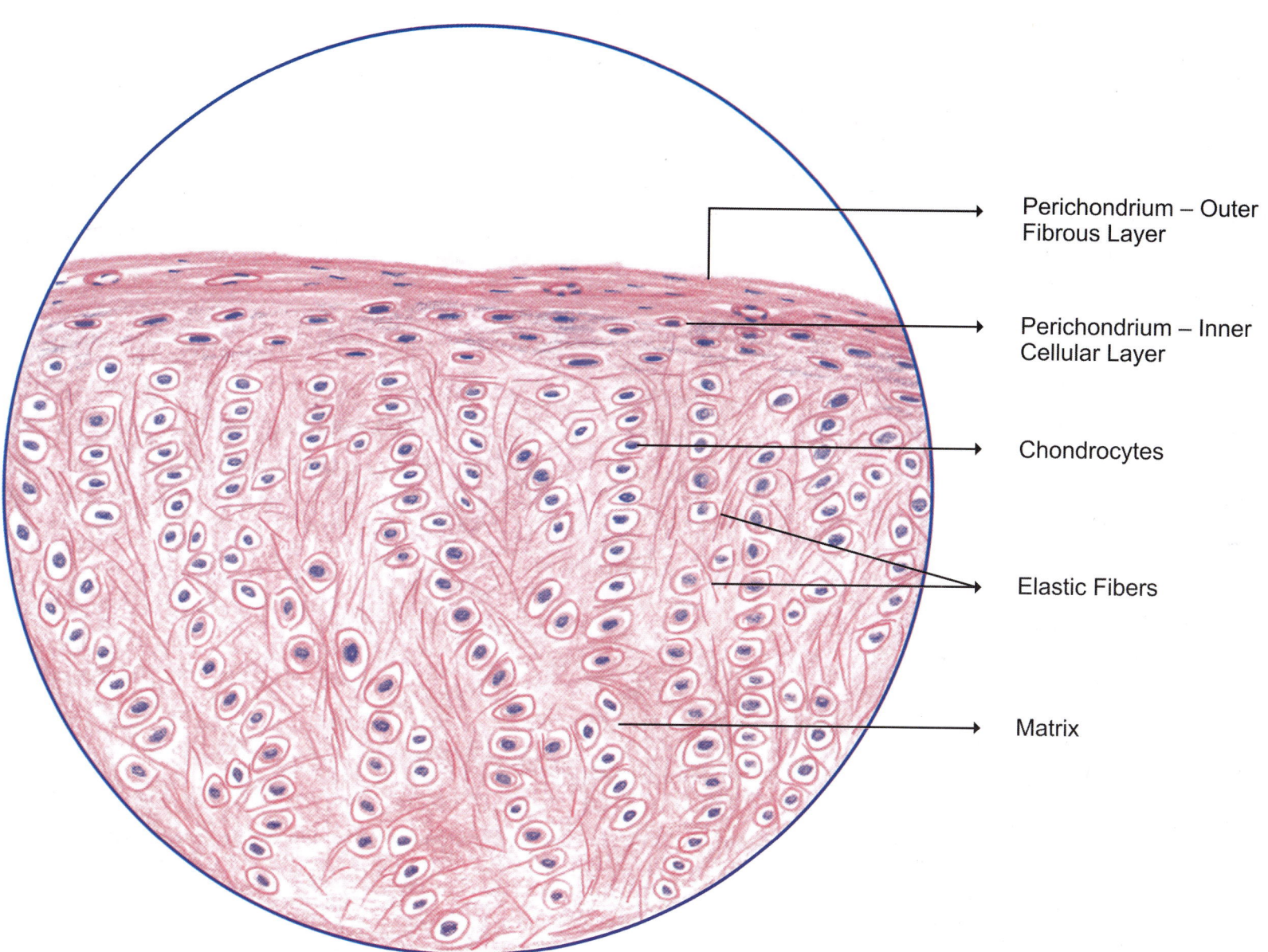

- Perichondrium – Outer Fibrous Layer
- Perichondrium – Inner Cellular Layer
- Chondrocytes
- Elastic Fibers
- Matrix

8. WHITE FIBROCARTILAGE

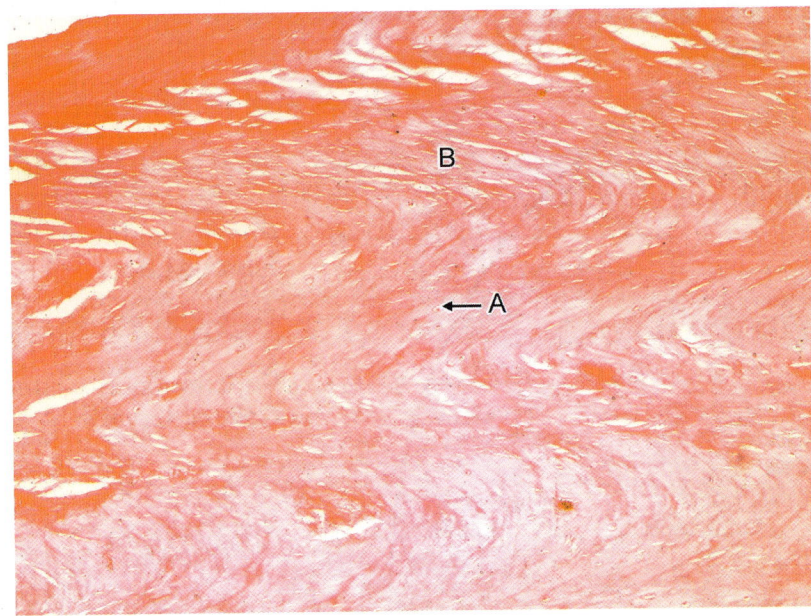

A	Chondrocytes in Rows
B	Bundles of Collagen Fibers

Identification Points
1. **Predominantly made of bundles of collagen fibers.**
2. **Scanty chondrocytes arranged in rows.**
3. **No perichondrium.**

- Chondrocytes are very few and small in size.
- Cells are arranged in rows located inside lacunae in between bundles of coarse collagen fibers.
- Perichondrium is absent.

Example: Intervertebral disc, cartilage of pubic symphysis, menisci of knee joint, articular disc of temporomandibular and sternoclavicular joints.

8. WHITE FIBROCARTILAGE

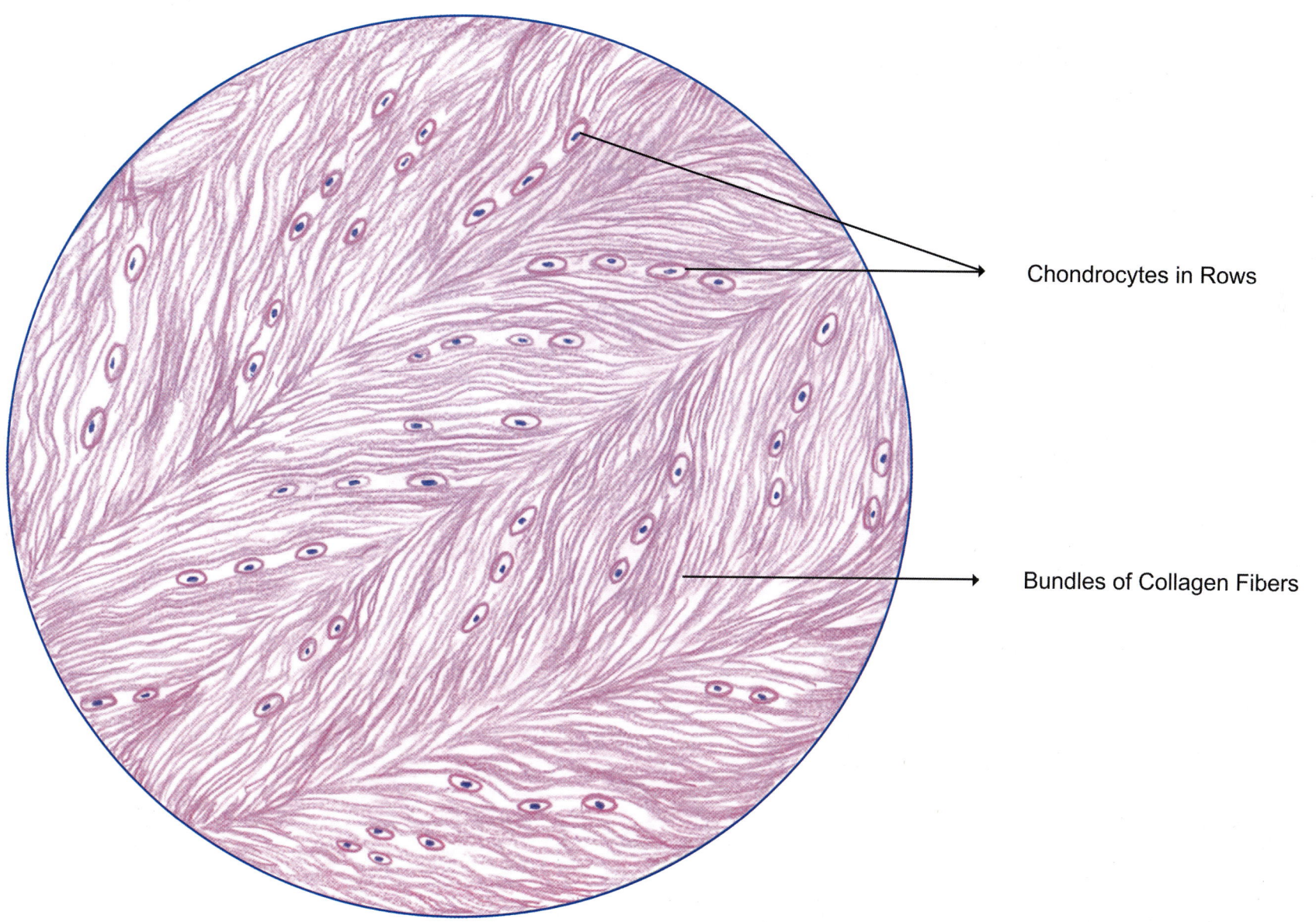

Chondrocytes in Rows

Bundles of Collagen Fibers

9. BONE—TRANSVERSE SECTION

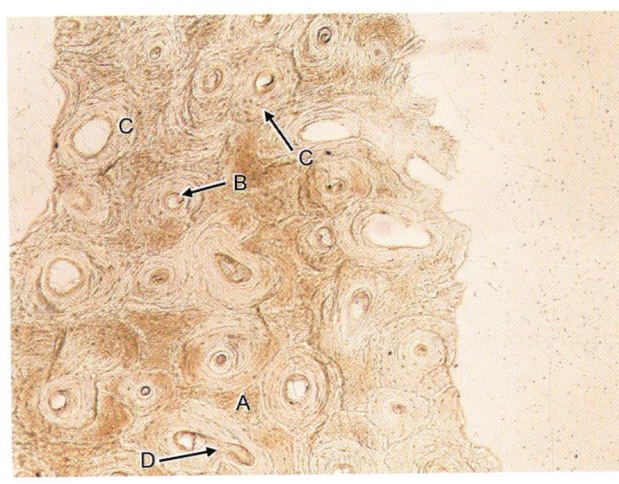

A	Interstitial Lamellae
B	Haversian Canal
C	Concentric Lamellae
D	Volkmann's Canal

Identification Points

1. **Transverse section of Haversian system with concentric lamellae around Haversian canal.**
2. **Lacunae containing osteocytes seen.**
3. **Circumferential and interstitial lamellae seen.**
4. **Periosteum present.**

- Haversian system is considered as the functional anatomical unit of bone.
- Haversian system or osteon is made up of central Haversian canal.
- Around the canal osteoid matrix is laid in layers called lamellae. Between the lamellae osteocytes are placed within the lacunae, which are interconnected by canaliculi. Lamellae around the canal are called concentric lamellae.
- At periphery running around the bone are circumferential lamellae which are located beneath the periosteum or endosteum.
- Lamellae between the Haversian system are called interstitial lamellae.
- Periosteum is a two-layered structure—outer fibrous and inner cellular layer.
- Fibrous layer containing collagen fibers.
- Inner cellular layer with osteoprogenitor cells helps in appositional growth/secondary healing.
- Three types of cells are seen in bone:
  a. Osteoblasts are bone-forming cells.
  b. Osteoclasts are seen at the sites of bone resorption.
  c. Osteocytes are older inactive cells, buried between layers of osteoid.

Matrix is made of ground substance, fibers and inorganic substance mainly calcium and phosphorus.

9. BONE—TRANSVERSE SECTION

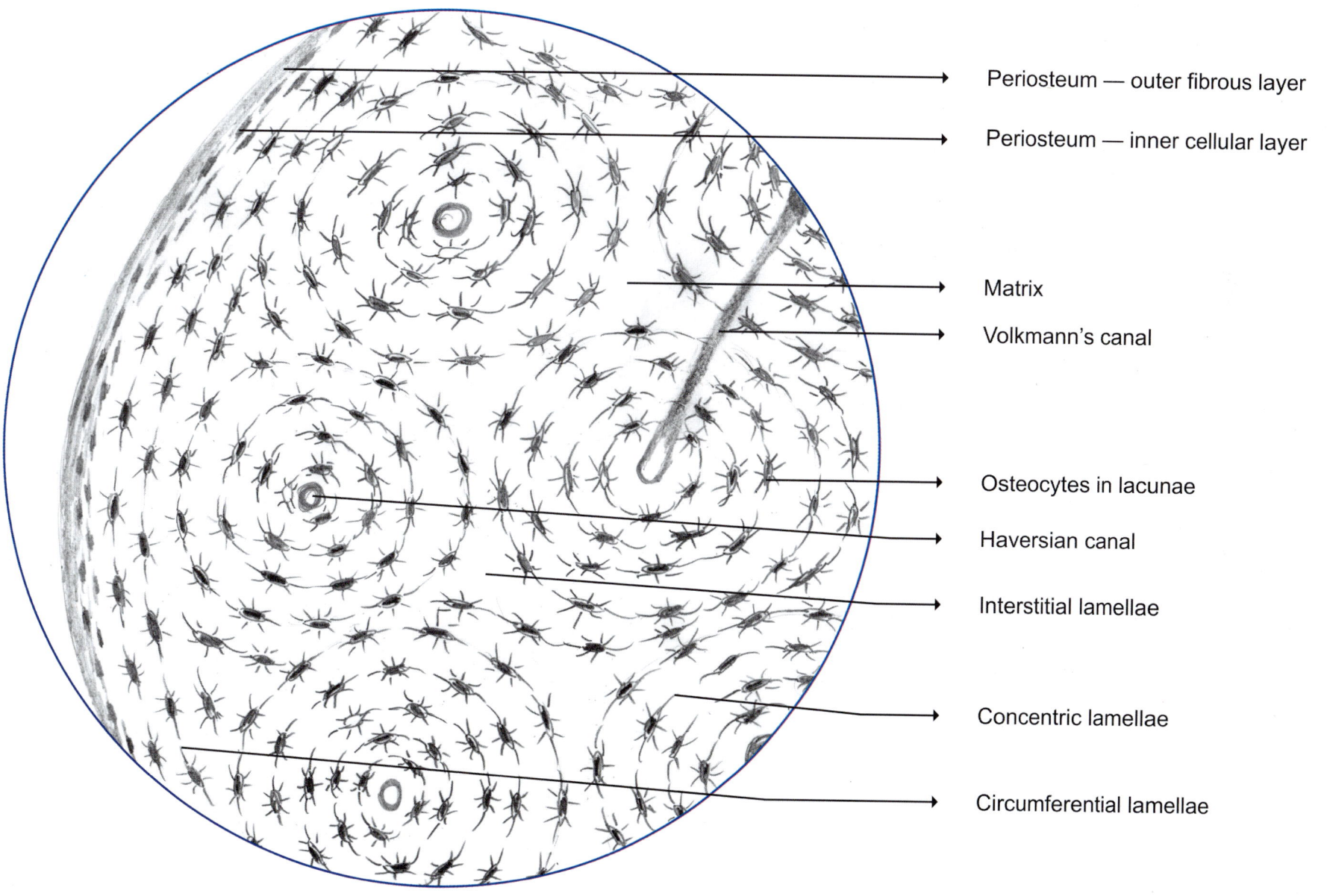

10. BONE—LONGITUDINAL SECTION

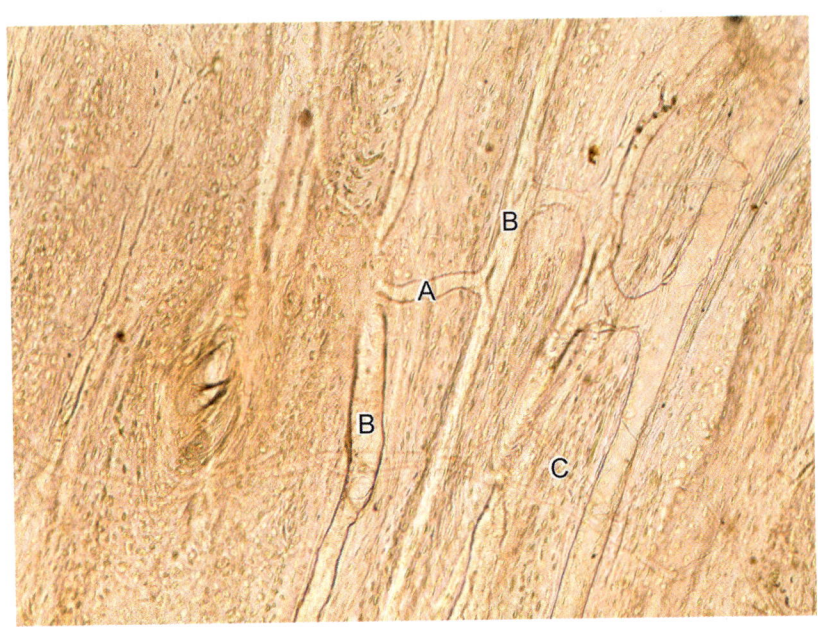

A	Volkmann's Canal
B	Haversian Canal
C	Osteocytes in Lacunae

Identification Points

1. **Longitudinal section of Haversian system with central Haversian canals.**
2. **Volkmann's canal—interconnecting the Haversian canals seen.**
3. **Lacunae containing osteocytes seen.**

- Haversian system is considered as the functional anatomical unit of bone.
- Haversian system or osteon is made up of central Haversian canal containing blood vessels and nerves.
- Around the canal, osteoid matrix is laid in layers called lamellae. Between the lamellae osteocytes are placed within the lacunae, which are interconnected by canaliculi.
- Haversian canals are interconnected by oblique canals called Volkmann's canals.
- At periphery running around the bone are circumferential lamellae which are located beneath the periosteum or endosteum.
- Periosteum is a two layered structure—outer fibrous and inner cellular layer.
  a. Fibrous layer containing collagen fibers
  b. Inner cellular layer with osteoprogenitor cells helps in appositional growth/secondary healing.

10. BONE—LONGITUDINAL SECTION

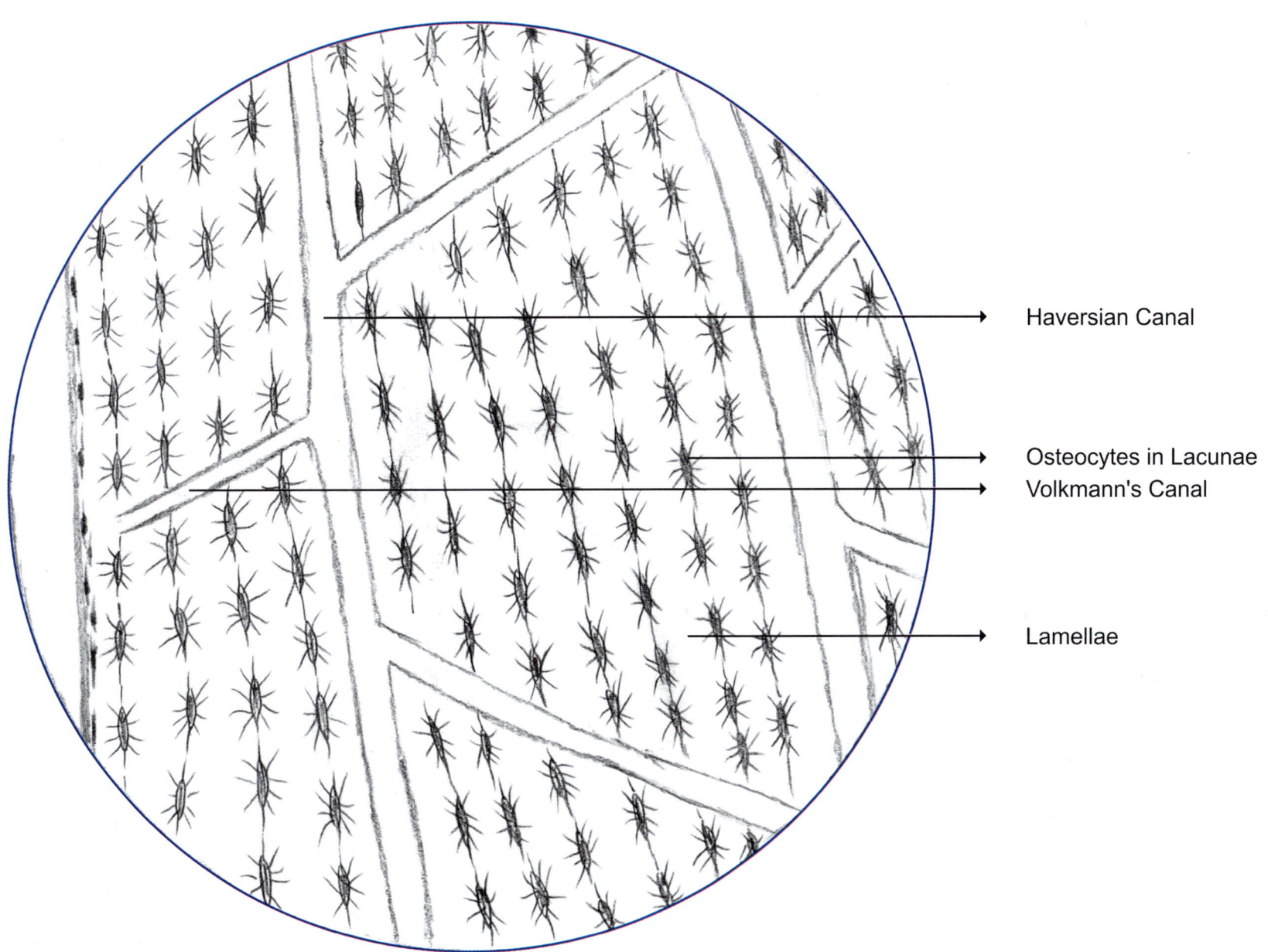

Haversian Canal

Osteocytes in Lacunae
Volkmann's Canal

Lamellae

11. CANCELLOUS BONE

Cancellous Bone

- Also called as spongy bone.
- It is made up of meshwork of irregularly-arranged trabeculae enclosing spaces which are filled by bone marrow and adipocytes.
- Each trabeculae contains many layers of lamellae separated by lacunae-containing osteocytes. Haversian system is not seen within trabeculae.
- The cytoplasmic processes of osteocytes radiate from the lacunae through the canaliculli.
- Endosteum lines the bony trabeculae, endosteal cells give rise to osteoblasts.

11. CANCELLOUS BONE

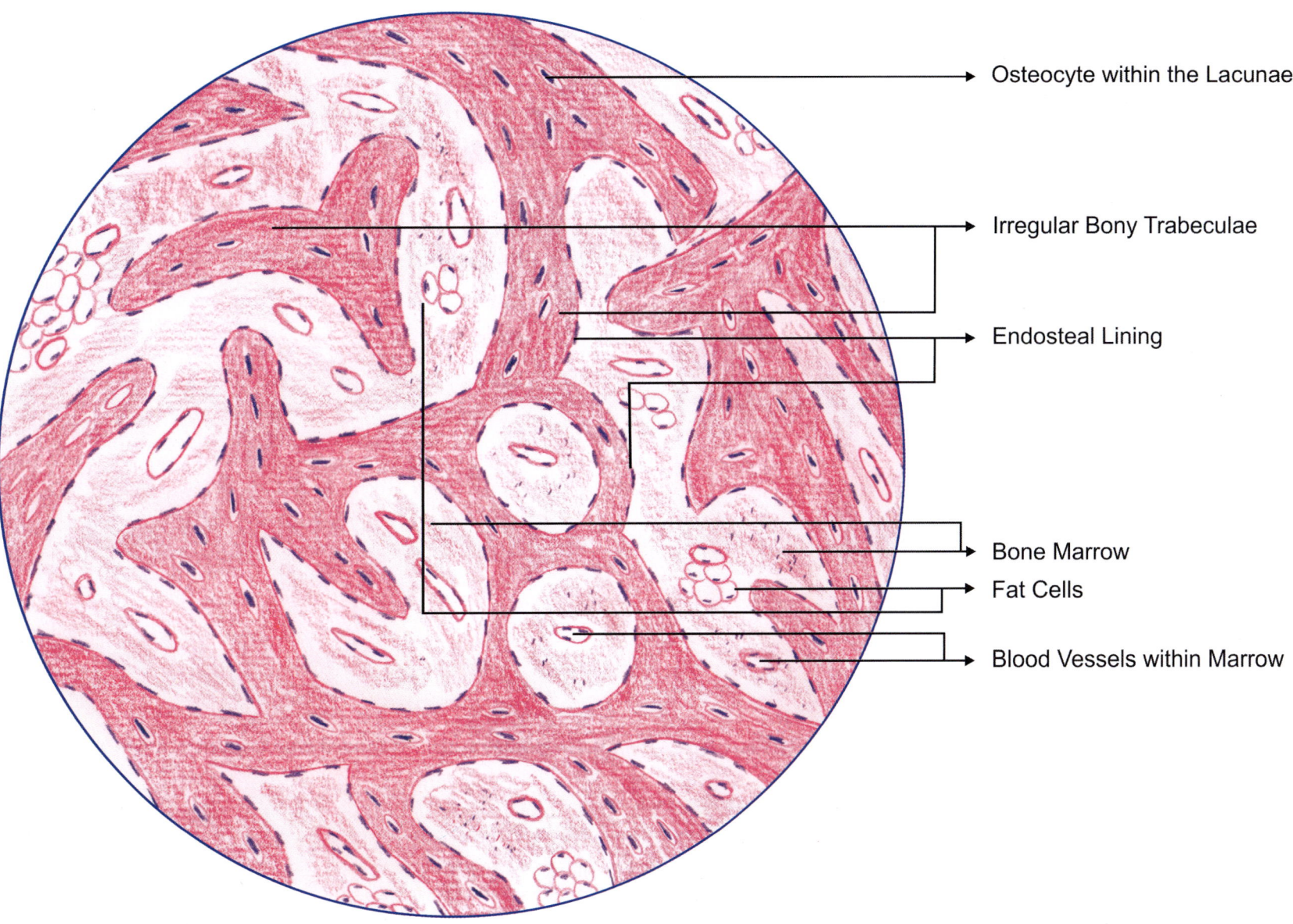

12. SKELETAL MUSCLE

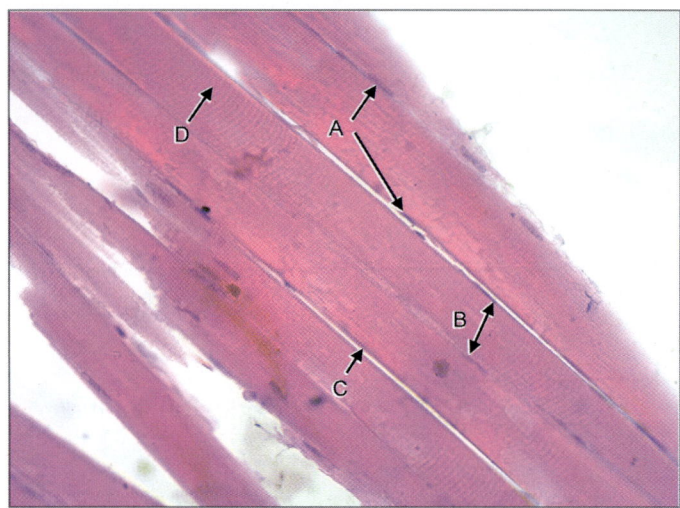

A	Peripheral Flat Nucleus
B	Muscle Fiber
C	Sarcolemma
D	Cross Striations

Identification Points

1. **Unbranched long cylindrical fibers.**
2. **Multiple peripherally placed flattened nuclei.**
3. **Dark and light cross striations seen.**

- Each cell is long cylindrical without branching.
- Fibers run parallel to each other.
- Skeletal muscles have transverse striations which are seen as light (I) and dark (A) bands. Hence they are called striated muscles. Striations are not easily seen under low magnification.
- Dark and light bands are due to regular arrangement of actin and myosin filaments.
- Center of 'I' band is called Z line. Center of 'A' band is light H zone. Dark M line is seen in the center of H zone.
- The part of myofibril between two adjacent Z lines is called sarcomere which is the functional unit of the muscle.
- 'A' band remains constant during muscle contraction, I and H bands become short.
- Skeletal muscle fiber or cell is covered by sarcolemma (cell membrane) and is multinucleated with flattened peripherally positioned nucleus.
- Skeletal muscles are voluntary muscles, innervated by somatic motor nerves.
- Connective tissue covering of each muscle fiber is endomysium. Bundles of such fibers (fascicles) are covered by perimysium. Entire muscle covered by epimysium.

12. SKELETAL MUSCLE

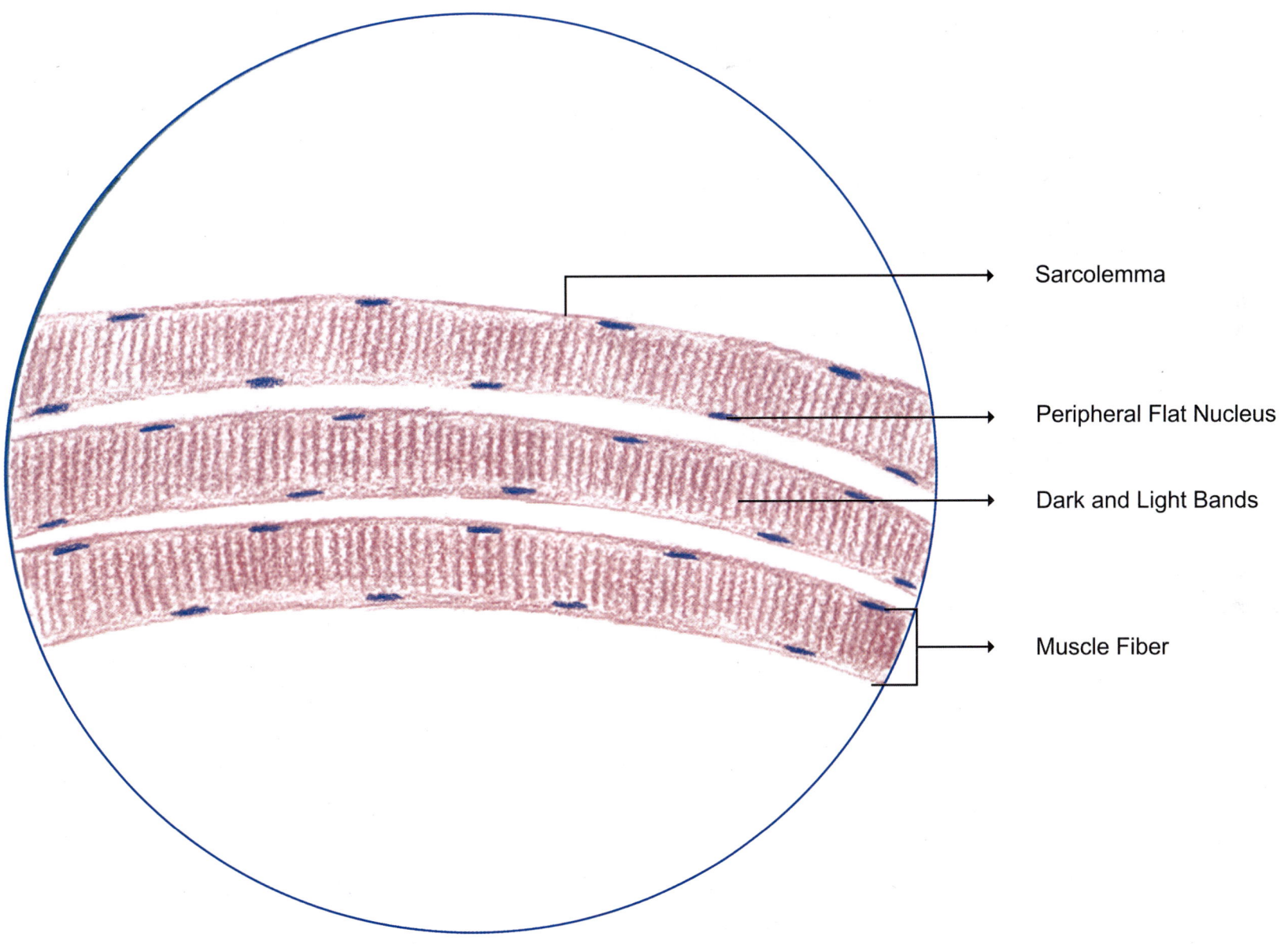

13. CARDIAC MUSCLE

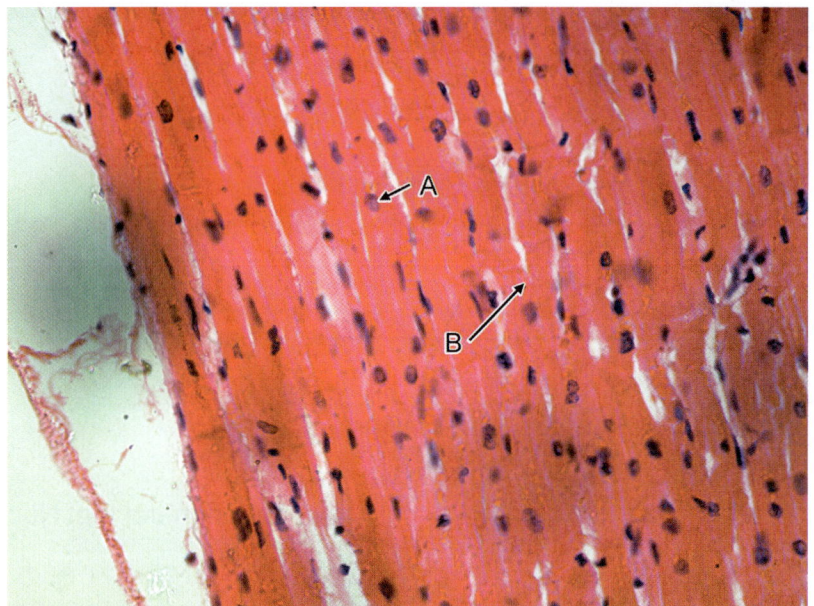

A	Single Centrally Placed Nucleus
B	Branching Cardiac Muscle Fiber

Identification Points

1. Short cylindrical fibers with central oval nuclei.
2. Branching of fibers seen.
3. Intercalated discs seen.

- Cardiac muscle fibers are small and cylindrical compared to skeletal muscle fibers.
- Nuclei are central, single and oval.
- Muscle fibers are branched.
- Intercalated disc one of the unique feature of cardiac muscle is the junction between adjacent cardiac muscle cells.
- It is zig zag in appearance and made up of three types of cell junctions—desmosomes, gap junctions and tight junctions. Allows electrical impulse to pass from one cell to another and makes the cardiac muscle fiber a functional syncytium.
- Cardiac muscle is also striated but striations are not prominent under lower magnification.
- Cardiac muscle is involuntary, seen only in heart.
- It is highly vascular and innervated by autonomic nervous system.

13. CARDIAC MUSCLE

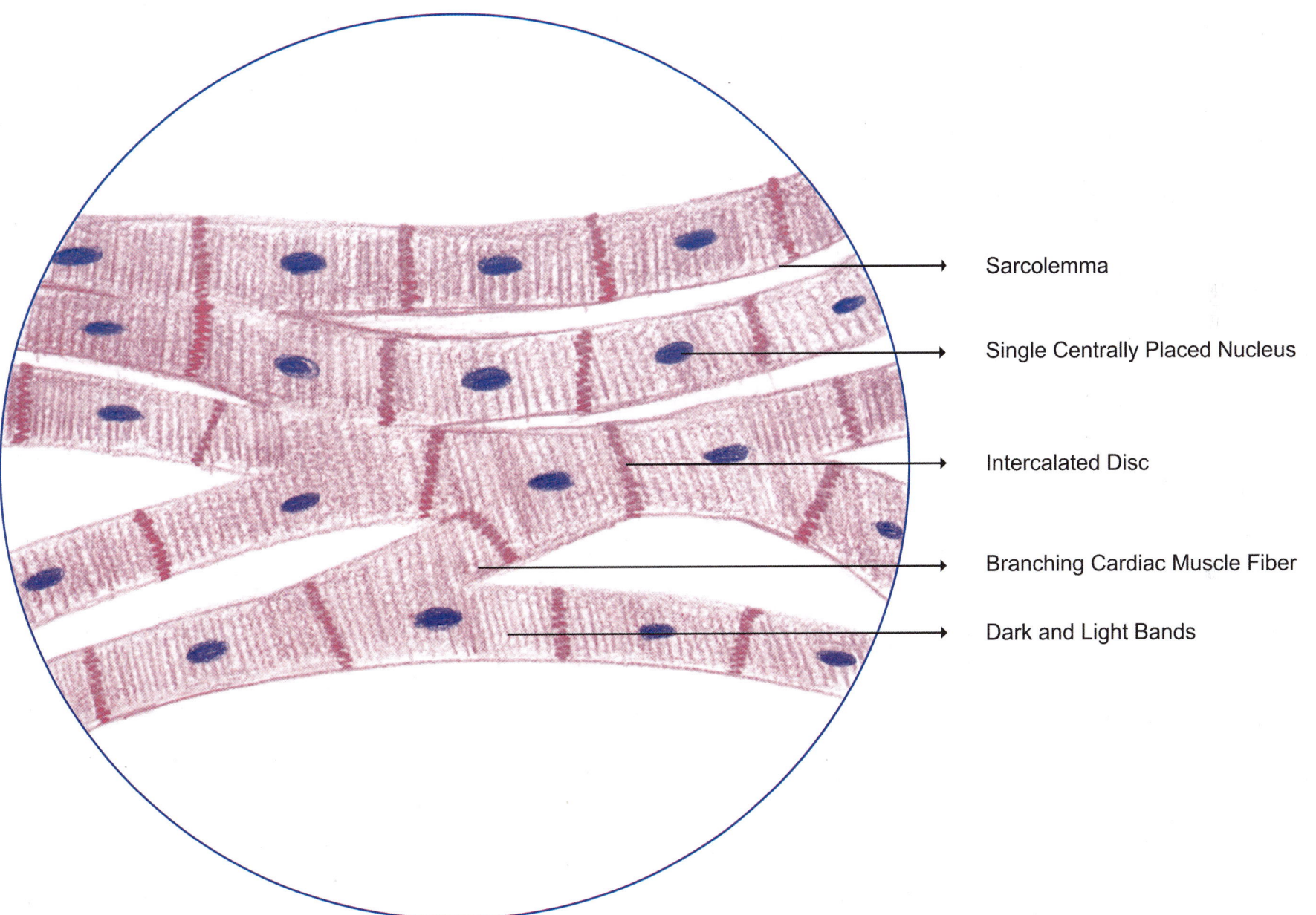

14. SMOOTH MUSCLE

Smooth Muscle

- Non-striated, involuntary.
- Spindle or fusiform-shaped cells with central oval-elongated nucleus.
- Sarcoplasm contains actin and myosin filaments without an orderly arrangement. Hence only longitudinal striations are seen.
- Found in walls of the digestive tracts, blood vessels, uterus, etc.
- Innervated by parasympathetic and sympathetic nerves.

14. SMOOTH MUSCLE

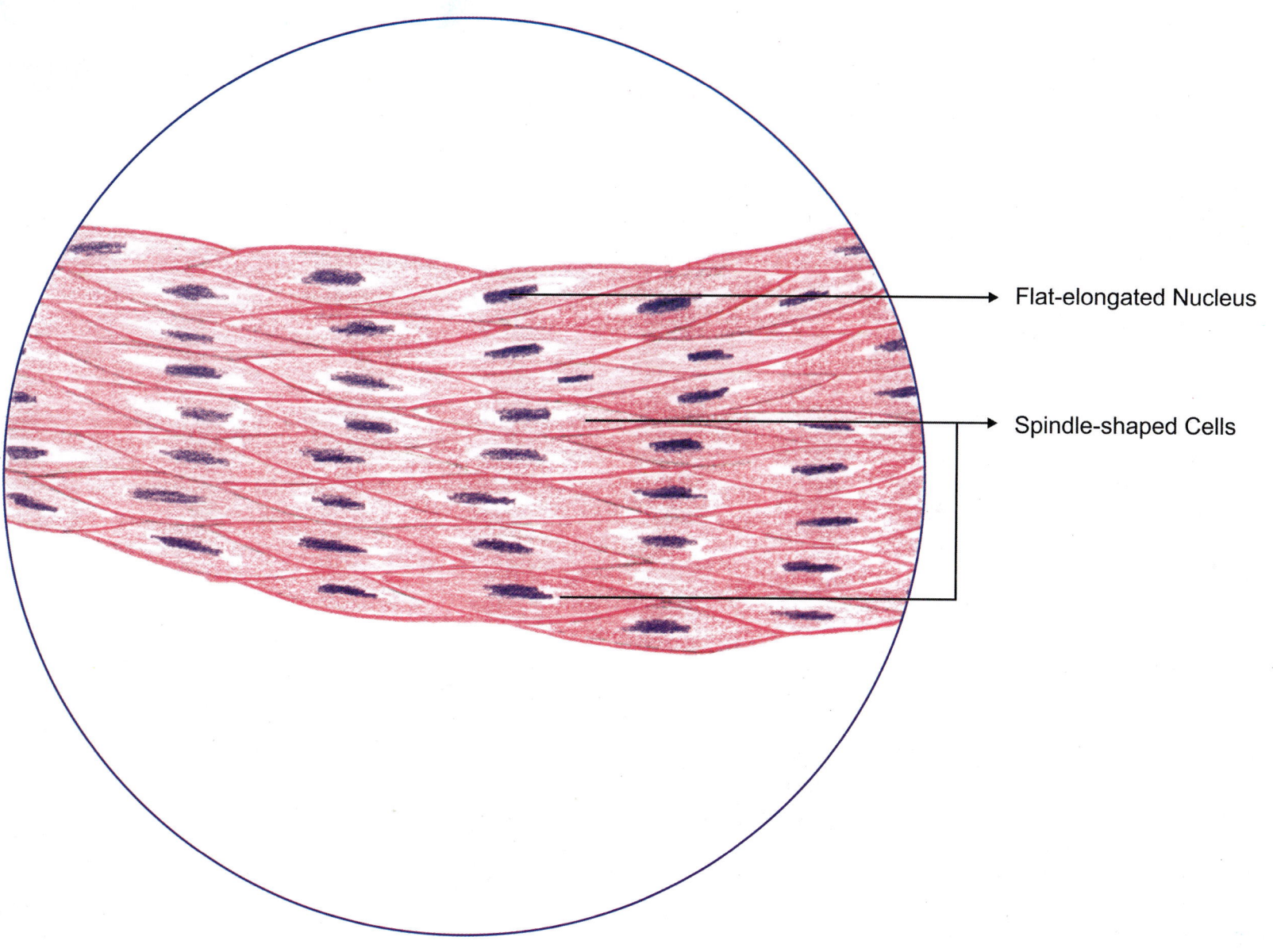

15. PERIPHERAL NERVE—TRANSVERSE SECTION

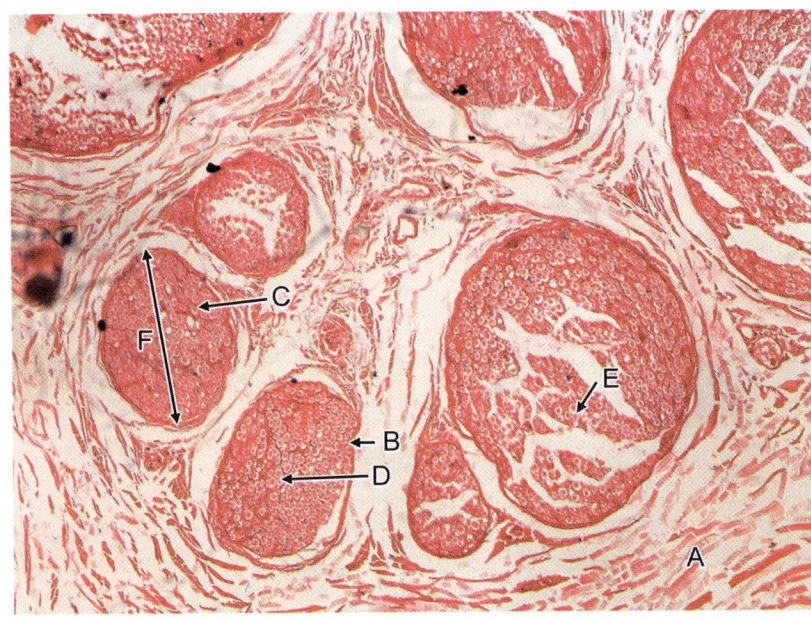

A	Epineurium
B	Perineurium
C	Endoneurium
D	Axons
E	Myelin Sheath
F	Fascicles

Identification Points

1. **Bundles of nerve fibers with connective tissue coverings.**
2. **Each myelinated axon surrounded by endoneurium.**
3. **Fascicles surrounded by perineurium.**
4. **Epineurium—outermost covering of nerve.**

- Peripheral nerves are formed by bundles of axons which may be myelinated or non-myelinated.
- Nerve fibers are surrounded by supporting cells called Schwann cells, forming a sheath called neurilemma.
- In myelinated nerve fibers the Schwann cell undergo spiraling around the axon forming the fatty myelin sheath whereas in unmyelinated fibers they only form the neurilemma.
- Part of axon between two adjacent Schwann cells not covered with myelin is called nodes of Ranvier, helps in fast conduction of impulses.
- Each myelinated axon is surrounded by connective tissue endoneurium.
- Fascicles of nerve fibers surrounded by perineurium.
- Outermost covering of nerve fiber is epineurium.

15. PERIPHERAL NERVE—TRANSVERSE SECTION

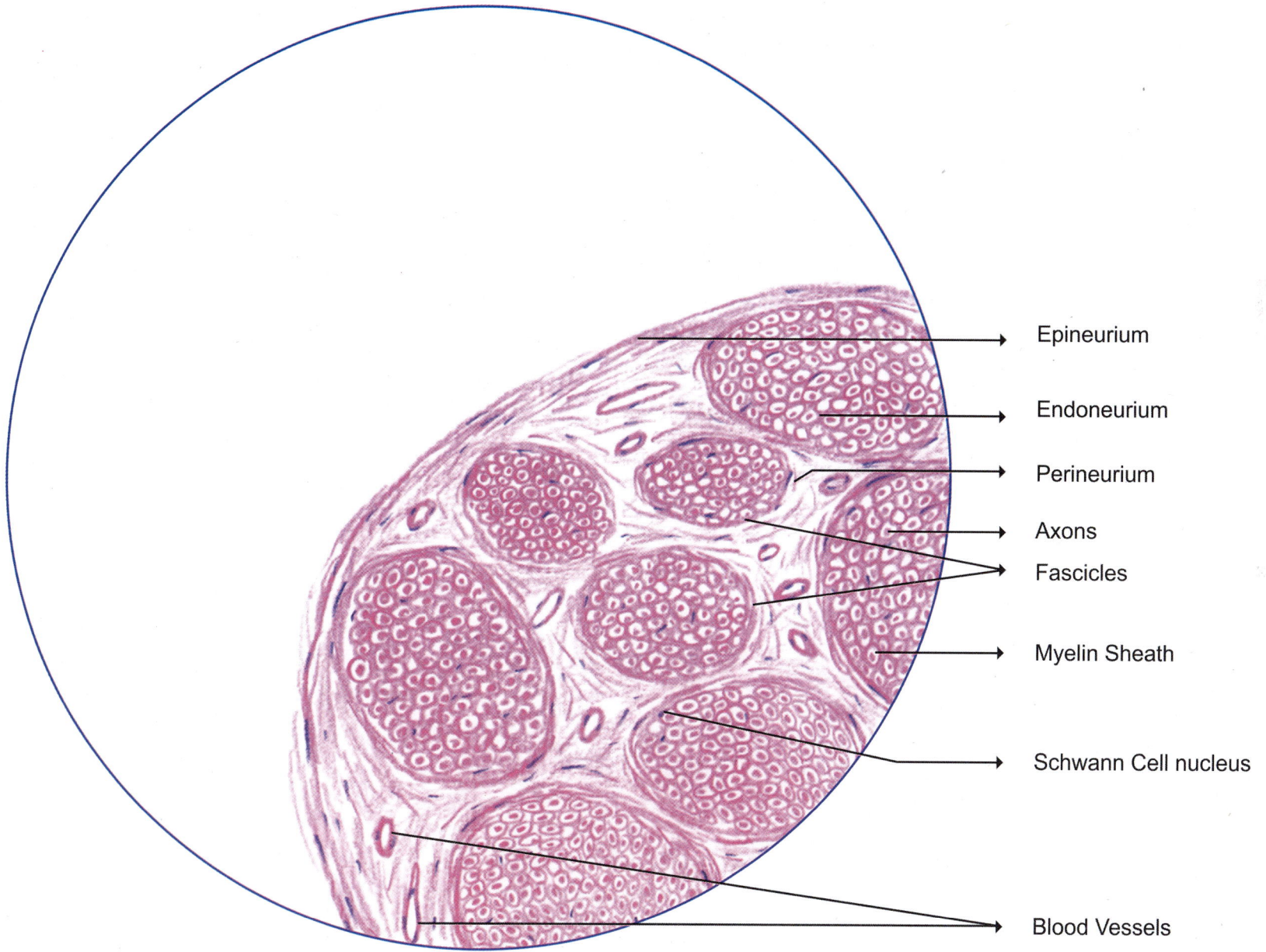

16. PERIPHERAL MYELINATED NERVE

Peripheral Myelinated Nerve

Peripheral myelinated nerve—transverse section and longitudinal section—osmic acid stain

1. **Bundles of nerve fibers seen.**
2. **In longitudinal section—thick black band of myelin sheath around light-stained axons seen. Nodes of Ranvier seen.**
3. **In transverse section—thick black ring of myelin sheath around unstained axons seen.**

- Each peripheral myelinated nerve fiber is surrounded by supporting cells called Schwann cells which undergo spiraling around the axon to form a fatty sheath called myelin sheath. It provides protection and insulation to the fiber.
- To illustrate the myelin sheath, a special stain, osmic acid is used. This stains the lipid in the myelin sheath black, whereas the axon remains unstained.
- In longitudinal section—the nerve fibers are seen as thick black band of myelin sheath around light-stained axons.
- Part of axon between two adjacent Schwann cells not covered with myelin is called nodes of Ranvier, helps in fast conduction of impulses.
- In transverse section—the nerve fibers appear as thick black ring of myelin sheath around unstained axons.
- Each myelinated axon is surrounded by connective tissue endoneurium.
- Fascicles of nerve fibers surrounded by perineurium.
- Outermost covering of nerve fiber is epineurium.

16. PERIPHERAL MYELINATED NERVE

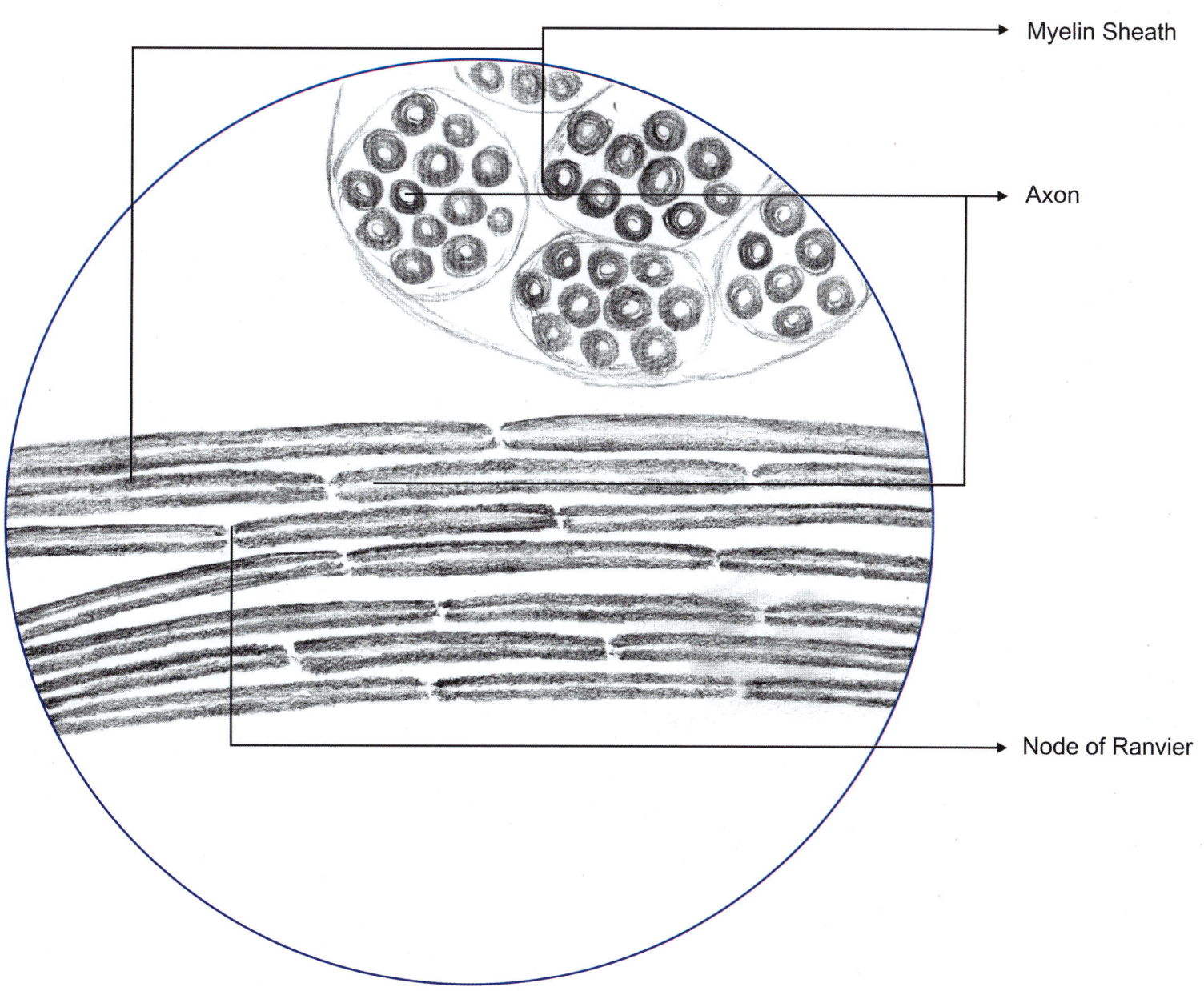

17. OPTIC NERVE—TRANSVERSE SECTION

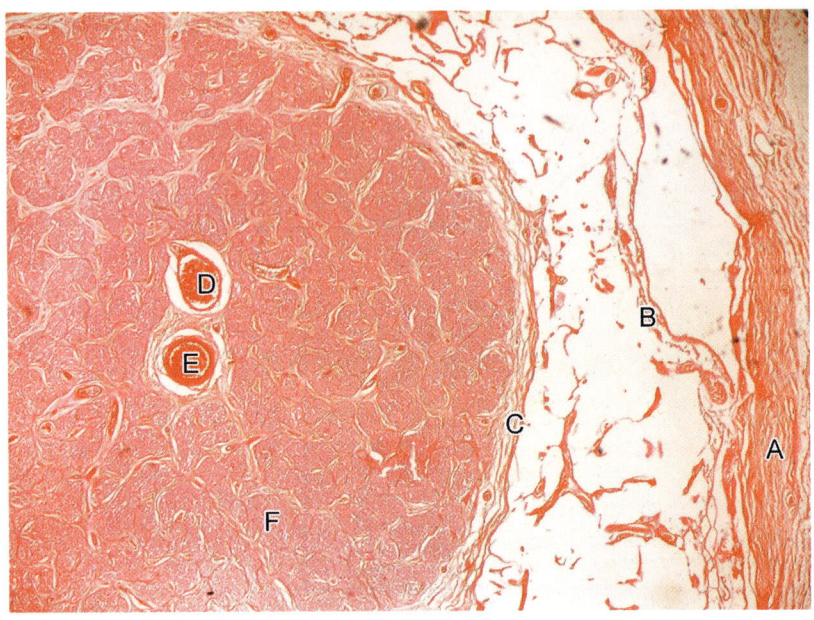

A	Dura Mater
B	Arachnoid Mater
C	Pia Mater
D	Central Vein of Retina
E	Central Artery of Retina
F	Bundles of Axons

Identification Points

1. **Myelinated axons grouped as bundles or fascicles.**
2. **In the center of the nerve, central artery and vein of retina are seen.**
3. **Shows three layers of meningeal coverings.**

- It is the second cranial nerve, a sensory nerve.
- Developmentally it is an outgrowth from brain.
- It has meningeal coverings similar to brain—dura mater, arachnoid, pia mater.
- Optic nerve contains myelinated axons of ganglion cells of retina.
- Axons grouped as bundles or fascicles by connective tissue extending from pia matter.
- Axons are myelinated by the oligodendrocytes.
- Central artery, branch of ophthalmic artery is an end-artery, is accompanied by central vein of retina.

17. OPTIC NERVE—TRANSVERSE SECTION

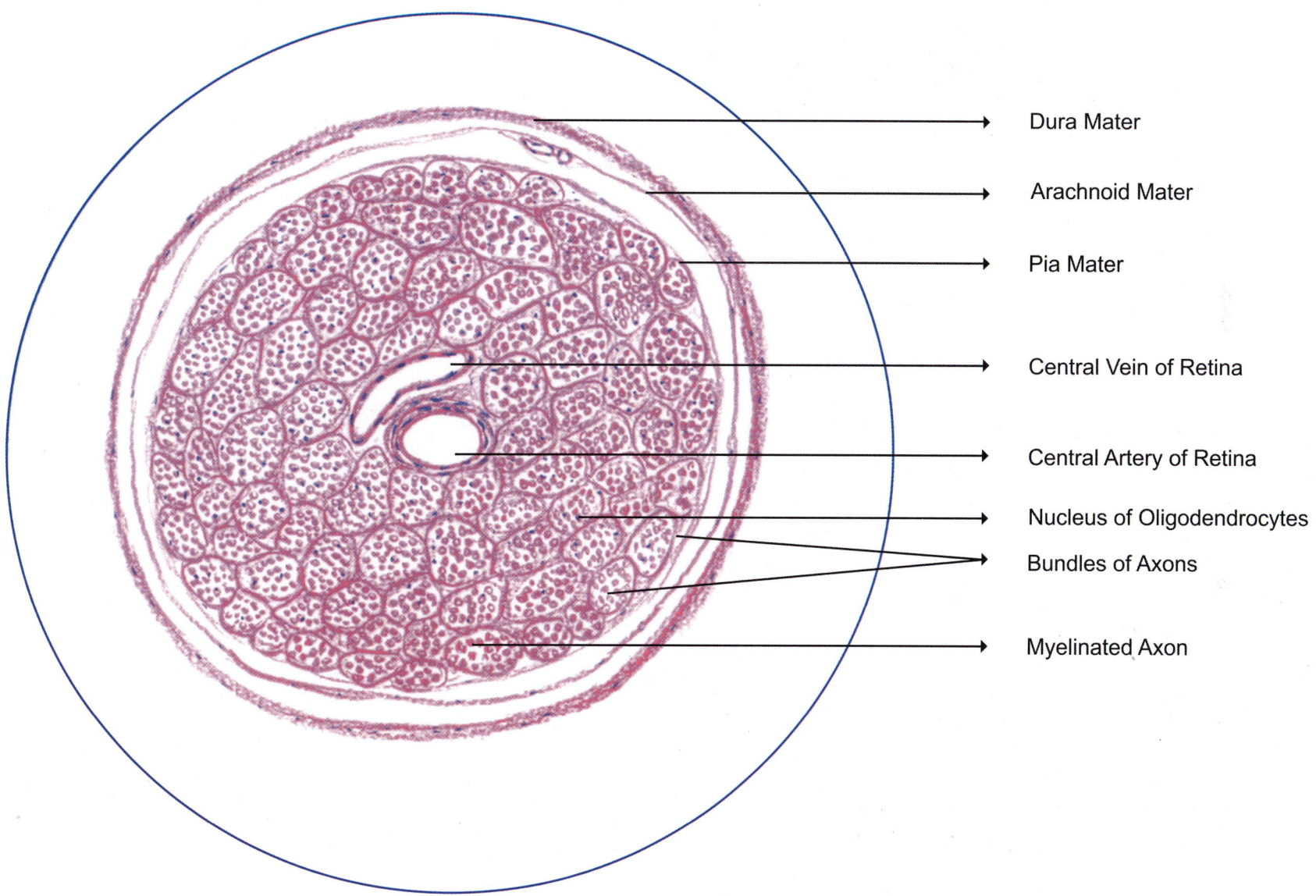

18. SYMPATHETIC GANGLION

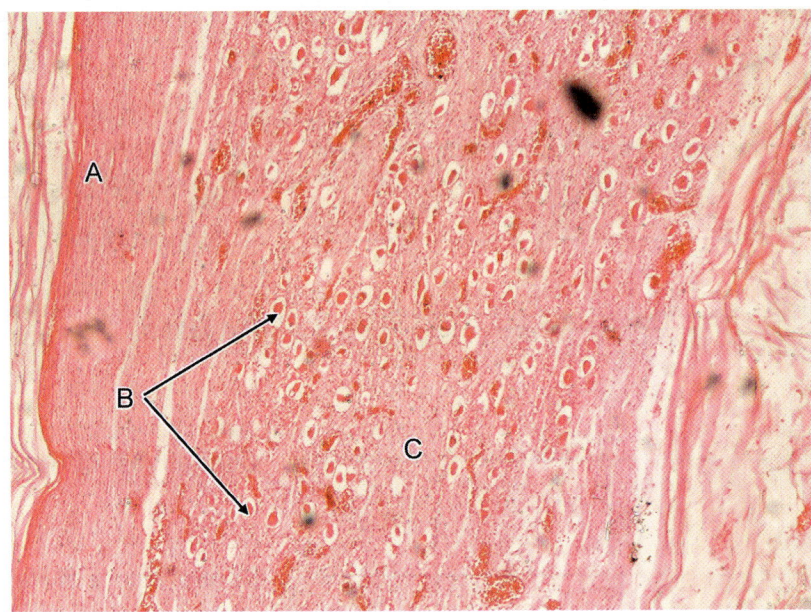

A	Capsule
B	Scattered Ganglion Cells
C	Nerve Fibers

Identification Points

1. **Small multipolar neurons with eccentric nucleus surrounded by satellite cells.**
2. **Scattered between the nerve fibers.**
3. **Thin connective tissue capsule.**

- Located in sympathetic trunk.
- Belong to autonomic nervous system, contains cell bodies of postganglionic sympathetic neurons.
- Thin connective tissue capsule present.
- Multipolar ganglion cells—small in size, with eccentric nucleus. Scattered between nerve fibers.
- Few satellite cells surround the ganglion cells and helps in nourishment and insulation.

18. SYMPATHETIC GANGLION

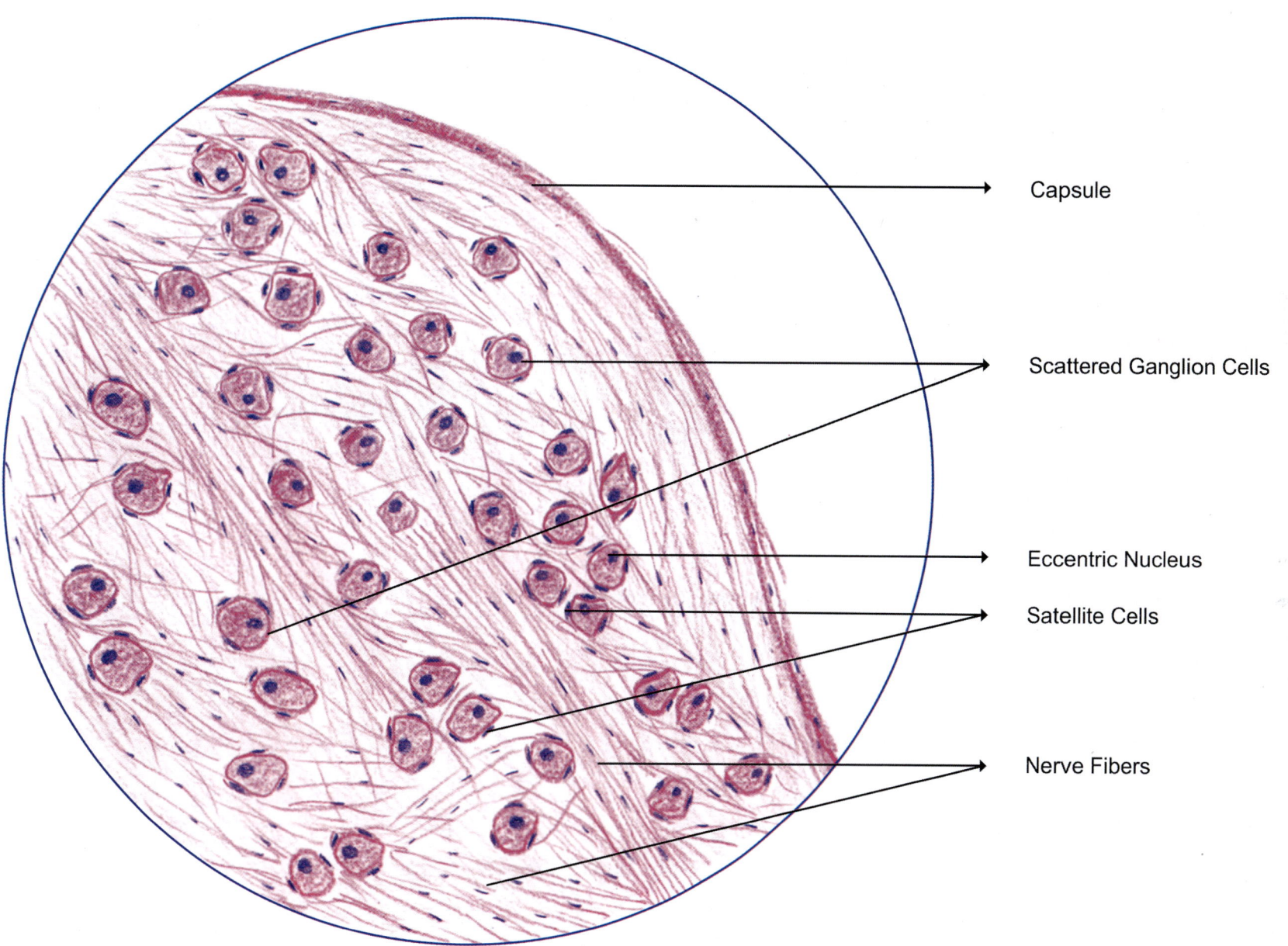

19. DORSAL ROOT GANGLION/SPINAL GANGLION

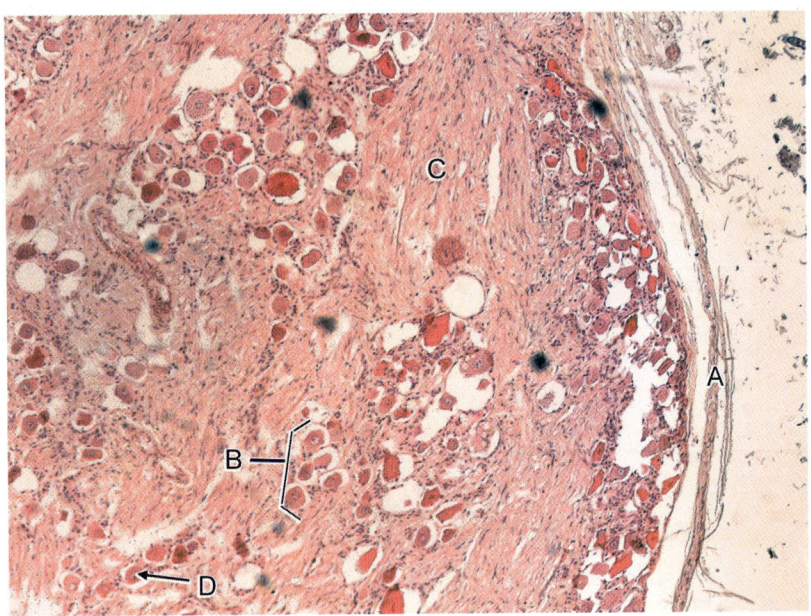

A	Capsule
B	Ganglion Cells in Groups
C	Nerve Fiber Bundles
D	Central Nucleus

Identification Points

1. Large pseudounipolar neurons with central nucleus surrounded by satellite cells.
2. Arranged in groups between bundles of nerve fibers.
3. Thick connective tissue capsule.

- They are also called as sensory ganglion.
- Present in dorsal root of spinal nerve.
- Contains first order sensory neurons.
- Thick connective tissue capsule seen.
- Pseudounipolar ganglion cells—large cells with central nucleus, arranged in groups.
- Satellite cells are more prominent forming a capsule around ganglion cells. It helps in nourishment and insulation.
- Bundles of parallel running myelinated and unmyelinated nerve fibers seen.

19. DORSAL ROOT GANGLION/SPINAL GANGLION

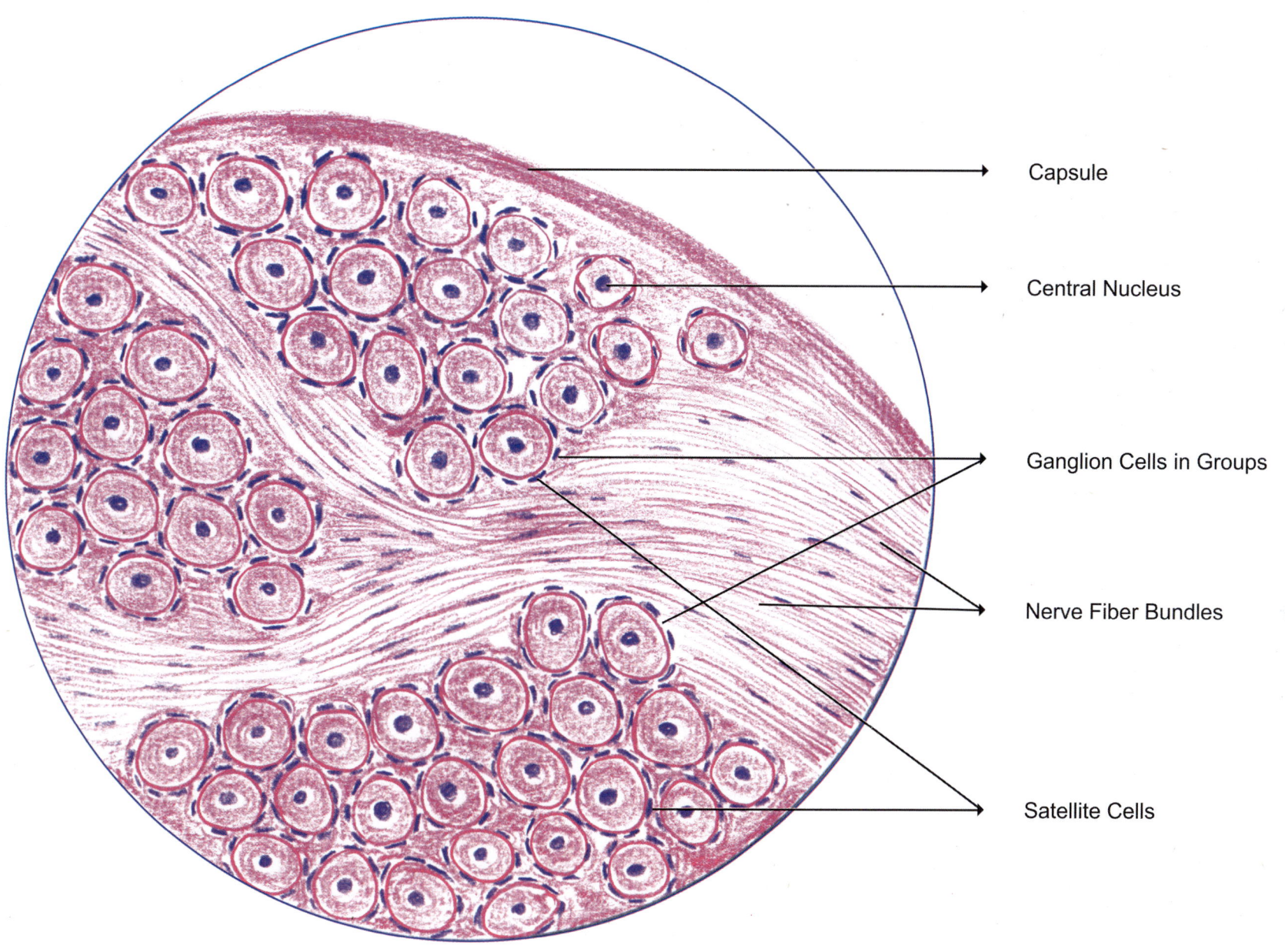

20. LARGE ARTERY/ELASTIC ARTERY

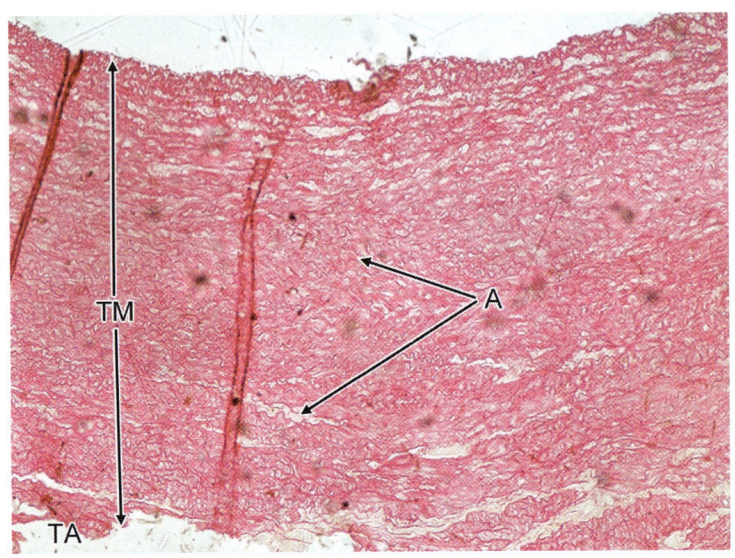

TM	Tunica Media
TA	Tunica Adventitia
A	Elastic Fibers

Identification Points

1. **Three layers of blood vessel—tunica intima, tunica media, tunica adventitia (externa).**
2. **Tunica media is thickest with more elastic fibers.**

1. **Tunica intima is the innermost layer, contains:**
   – Endothelium—flat squamous cells lines the lumen.
   – Subendothelial connective tissue.
   – Internal elastic lamina made of elastic fibers in the form of fenestrated membrane—not prominent.
2. **Tunica media—thickest layer:**
   – Elastic fibers are prominent in the form of concentric fenestrated lamellae. Hence, internal elastic lamina is not prominent. Help in recoil of the artery after distention.
   – Few smooth muscles fibers are also present.
   – Outer external elastic lamina present.
3. **Tunica adventitia:**
   – Outer most connective tissue layer with predominant collagen fibers. Also contains vasa vasorum (blood vessels that supply the walls of large blood vessels).

Example: Aorta, brachiocephalic trunk, common carotid, subclavian and common iliac arteries.

20. LARGE ARTERY/ELASTIC ARTERY

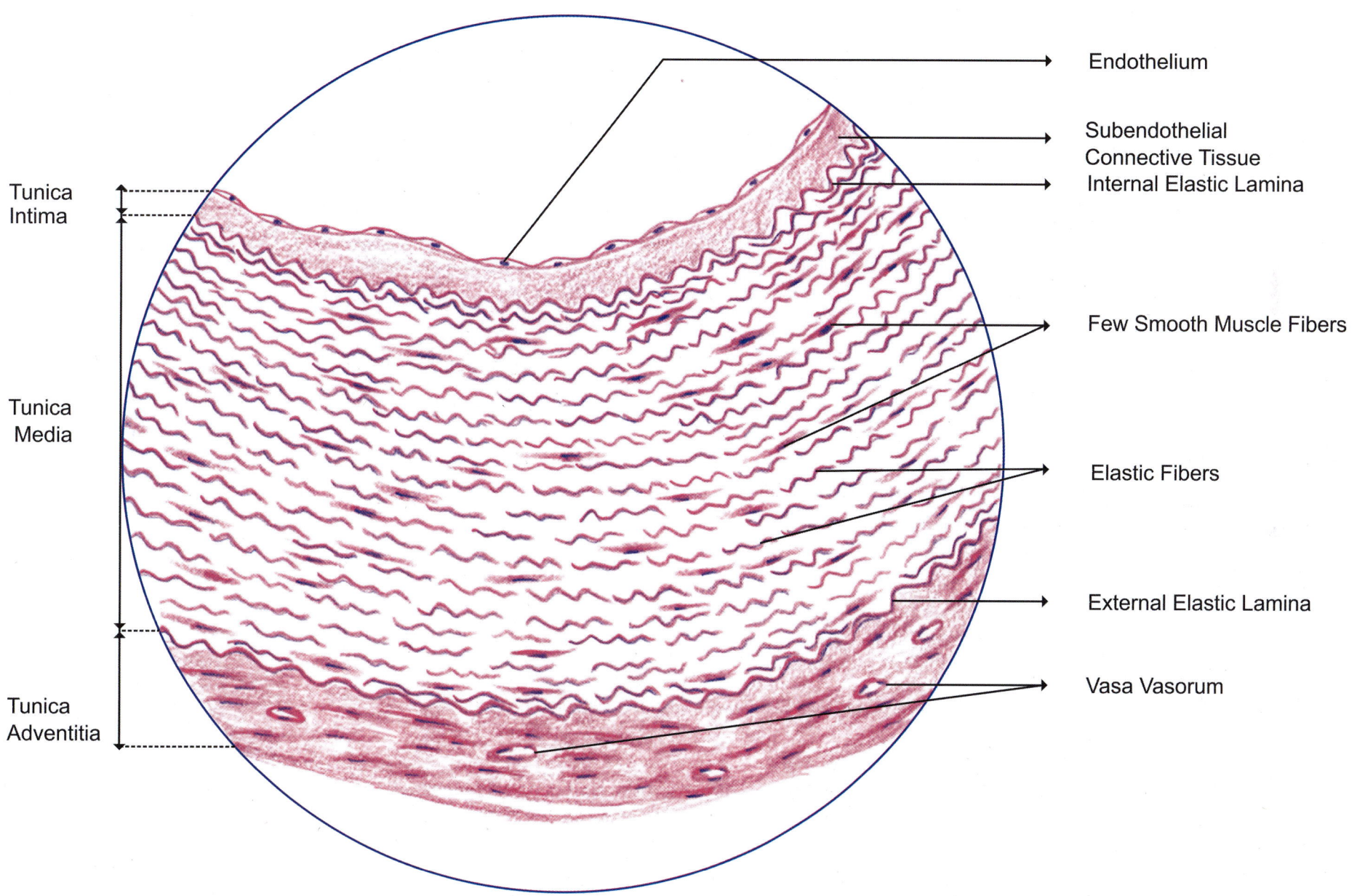

21. MEDIUM-SIZED ARTERY/MUSCULAR ARTERY

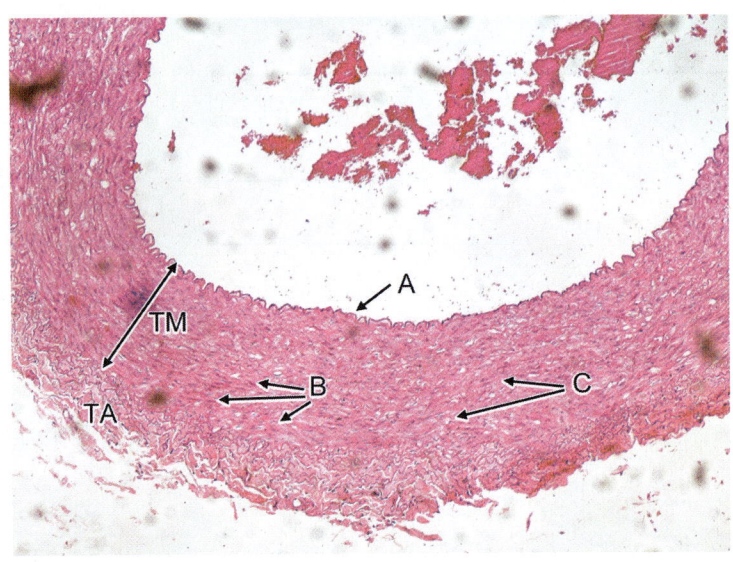

TM	Tunica Media
TA	Tunica Adventitia
A	Internal Elastic Lamina
B	Smooth Muscle Fibers
C	Few Elastic Fibers

Identification Points

1. Three layers of blood vessel—tunica intima, tunica media, tunica adventitia (externa).
2. Tunica media is thickest with more smooth muscle fibers.
3. Internal elastic lamina is prominent.

Made of three layers:

1. **Tunica intima is the innermost layer, contains:**
   - Endothelium—flat squamous cells lines the lumen.
   - Subendothelial connective tissue.
   - Internal elastic lamina made of elastic fibers in the form of fenestrated membrane. It is wavy and prominent.
2. **Tunica media—thickest layer:**
   - Smooth muscle fibers are predominant, circularly/spirally arranged.
   - Contraction of smooth muscles reduces the luminal diameter. They also give rise to the elastic and collagen fibers. Help in repair of damaged endothelial cells.
   - Few elastic fibers present.
   - Outer external elastic lamina present.
3. **Tunica adventitia—outer most layer:**
   - Contains connective tissue with collagen and elastic fibers.

Example: Radial, ulnar, popliteal arteries.

21. MEDIUM-SIZED ARTERY/MUSCULAR ARTERY

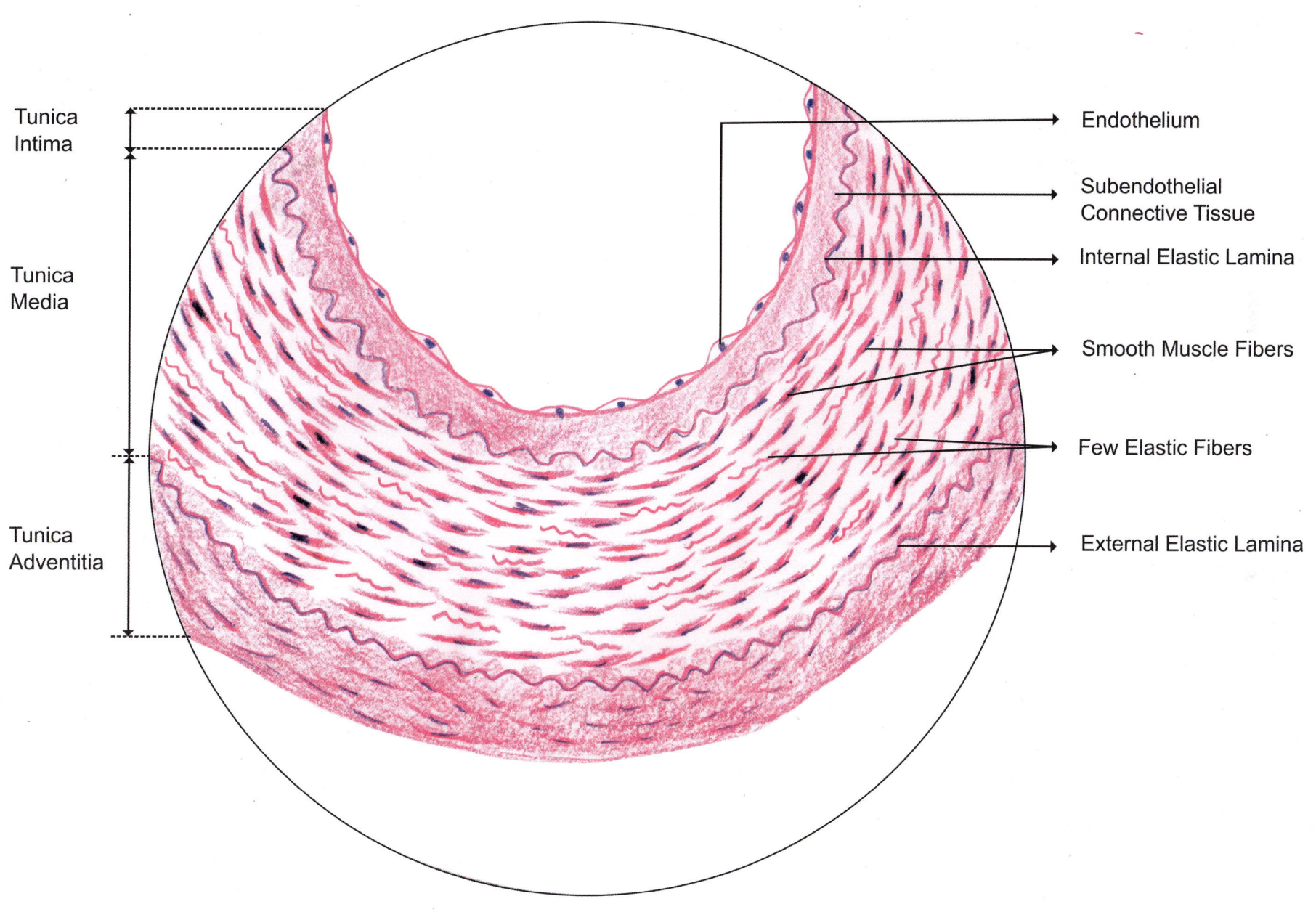

22. LARGE VEIN

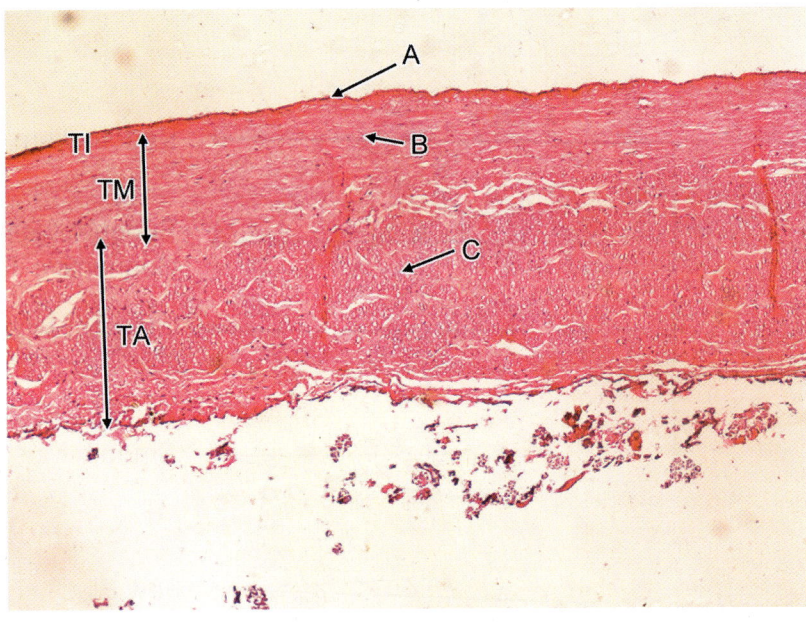

TI	Tunica Intima
TM	Tunica Media
TA	Tunica Adventitia
A	Endothelium
B	Smooth Muscle Fibers
C	Longitudinally Arranged Smooth Muscle Fibers

Identification Points

1. Three layers of blood vessel—tunica intima, tunica media, tunica adventitia (externa).
2. Tunica externa is thickest with smooth muscle fibers arranged in longitudinal bundles.

Made of three layers—not distinct, thin walled:

1. **Tunica intima—innermost layer, contains:**
   – Endothelium—flat squamous cells lines the lumen.
   – Subendothelial connective tissue and internal elastic lamina not well defined.
2. **Tunica media contains large amount of collagen fibers:**
   – Few smooth muscle fibers, elastic fibers present.
3. **Tunica adventitia—outer most layer, thickest layer:**
   – Connective tissue with collagen fibers.
   – Contains longitudinally running smooth muscle fibers.

Example: Inferior vena cava, superior vena cava.

22. LARGE VEIN

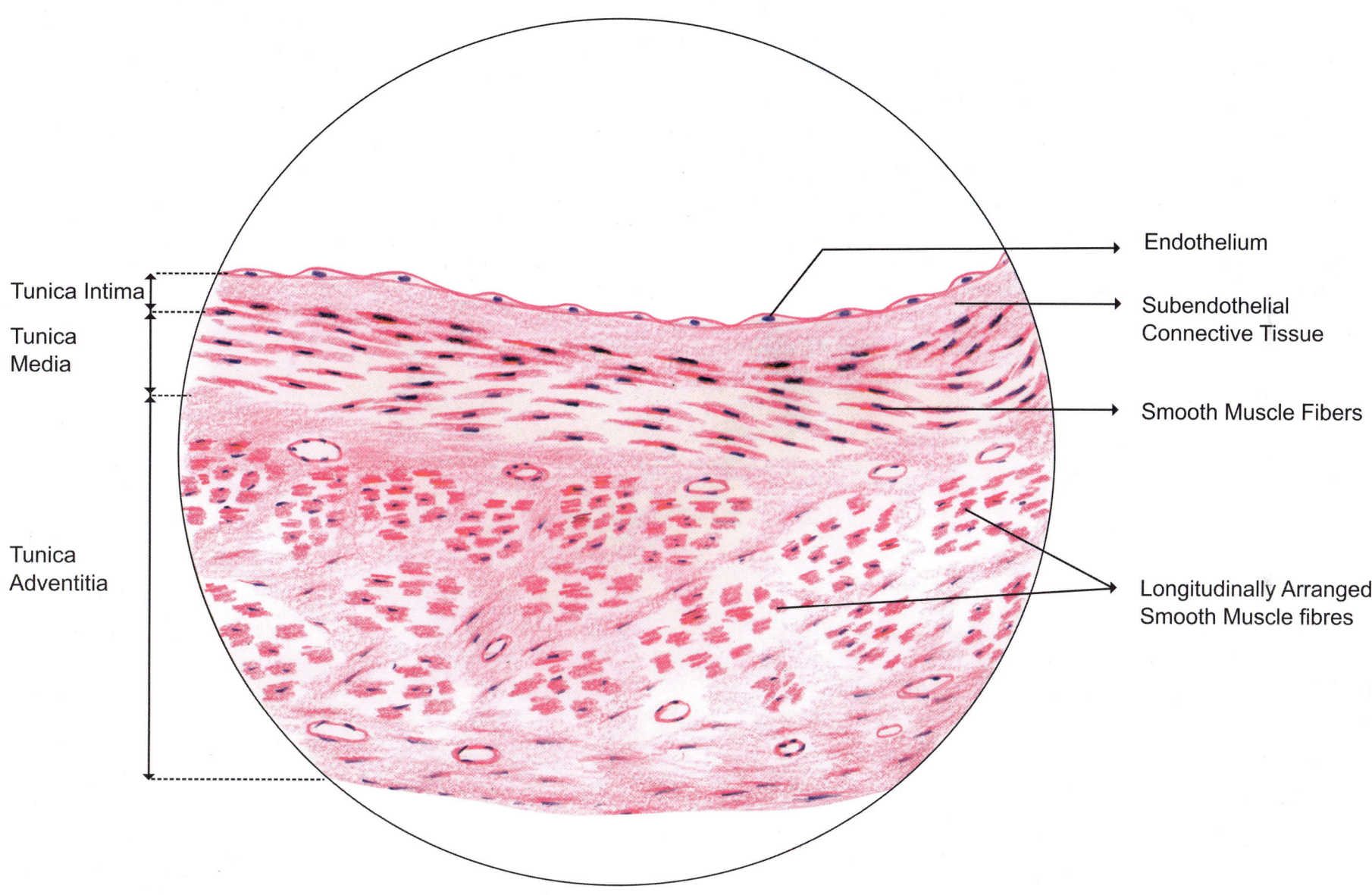

23. MEDIUM-SIZED VEIN

Medium-sized Vein

1. Three layers of blood vessel—tunica intima, tunica media, tunica adventitia (externa).
2. Tunica externa is thickest.

Made of three layers—not distinct, thin walled, collapsed lumen:
Diameter of more than 1 mm up to 10 mm, contains valves which are reduplication of endothelium.

1. **Tunica intima—innermost layer, contains:**
   - Endothelium—flat squamous cells with basal lamina lines the lumen,
   - Thin subendothelial connective tissue seen and internal elastic lamina not well defined.
2. **Tunica media:**
   - Contains both circular and longitudinal smooth muscle fibers, collagen fibers and Elastic fibers.
3. **Tunica adventitia:**
   - Outer most layer, thickest layer.
   - Connective tissue with collagen fibers and elastic fibers.

Example: Cephalic vein, basilic vein.

23. MEDIUM-SIZED VEIN

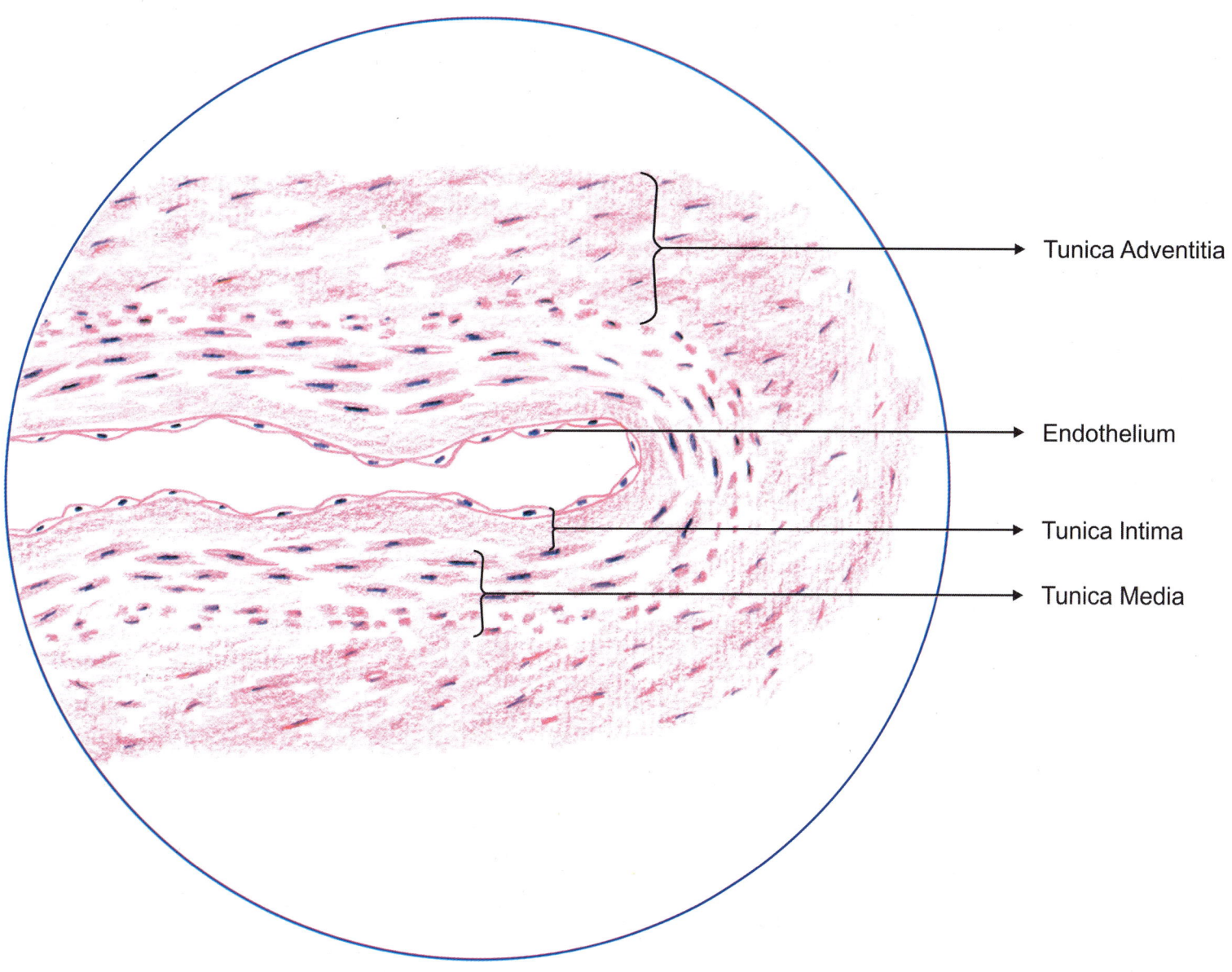

24. CAPILLARIES AND SINUSOIDS

Capillaries and Sinusoids

These are exchange vessels.

Capillary:
- Smallest diameter, 7–8 µm.
- Each capillary lined by simple-flattened cells on a basal lamina. They have flat nucleus.
- Perivascular cells called pericytes may be seen, which may help in phagocytosis and growth of new capillaries.

Types
1. Continuous—present in most parts of body like skin, brain, lungs.
2. Fenestrated—have pores between the endothelial cells, seen in endocrine glands and renal corpuscles.

Sinusoids
- Are dialated, tortuous vessels of about 20 µm diameter with incomplete walls and irregular lumen.
- Have sluggish blood flow, blood comes in direct contact with tissue cells.
- Lined by flat endothelial cells with thin layer of connective tissue.
- Found in liver, adrenal cortex, pituitary, spleen, bone marrow.

24. CAPILLARIES AND SINUSOIDS

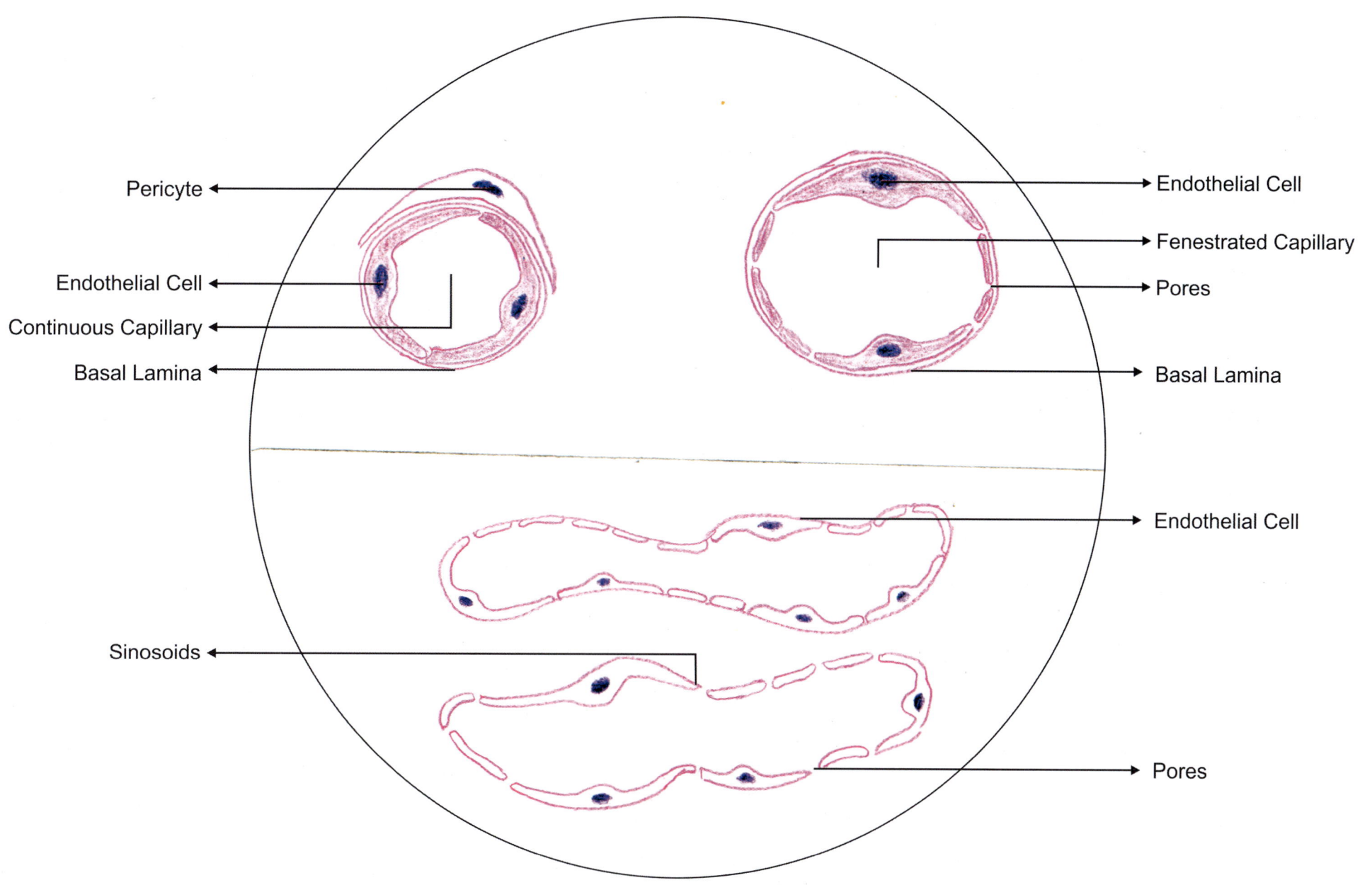

25. LYMPH NODE

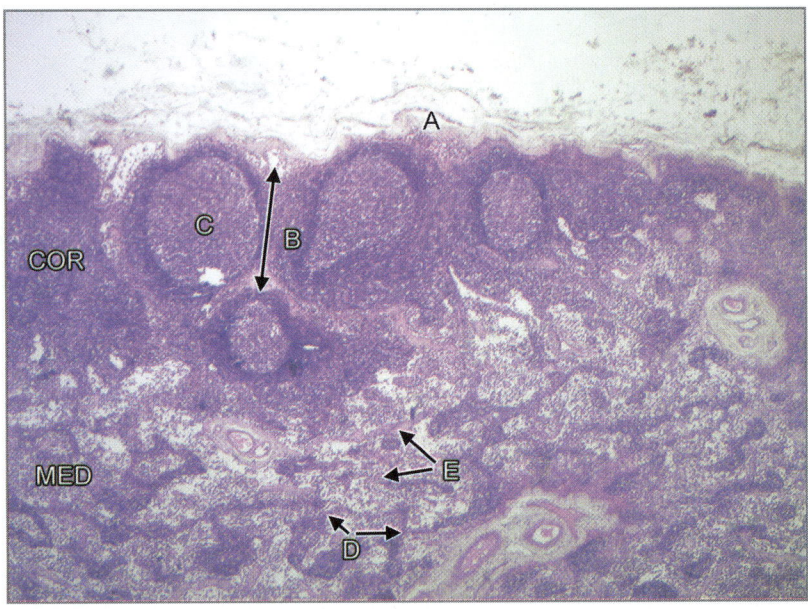

COR	Cortex
MED	Medulla
A	Capsule
B	Lymphoid Follicle
C	Germinal Center
D	Medullary Cords
E	Medullary Sinus

Identification Points

1. **Fibrous capsule and subcapsular space seen.**
2. **Outer cortex, inner medulla differentiated.**
   Cortex contains lymphoid follicles with germinal center.
   Medulla contains medullary cords and sinuses.

- Lymph node has outer fibrous capsule. This sends trabeculae inside. There is distinct subcapsular space.
- Afferent lymphatics around the gland pierces the capsule and drain into subcapsular space.
- Cortex contains lymphoid follicles with pale staining germinal center. Rim of the follicles have densely packed inactive B lymphocytes. Germinal centers contain pale staining large, rapidly dividing B lymphocytes.
- Paracortex, which is the junction between cortex and medulla contains T lymphocytes.
- In medulla lymphocytes arranged like branching cords along the sinuses called as medullary cords. These are mainly macrophages and plasma cells.
- Lymph will drain from the afferent lymphatics into subcapsular sinus, then passes along the trabacular sinus into medullary sinuses.
- Finally drains out from the hilum through the efferent lymphatics.
- As it passes through the sinuses it comes in contact with antigen presenting cells which present it to the lymphocytes.
- Functions of lymph node—filtration of lymph, proliferation of lymphocytes and forms a part of immune system.

25. LYMPH NODE

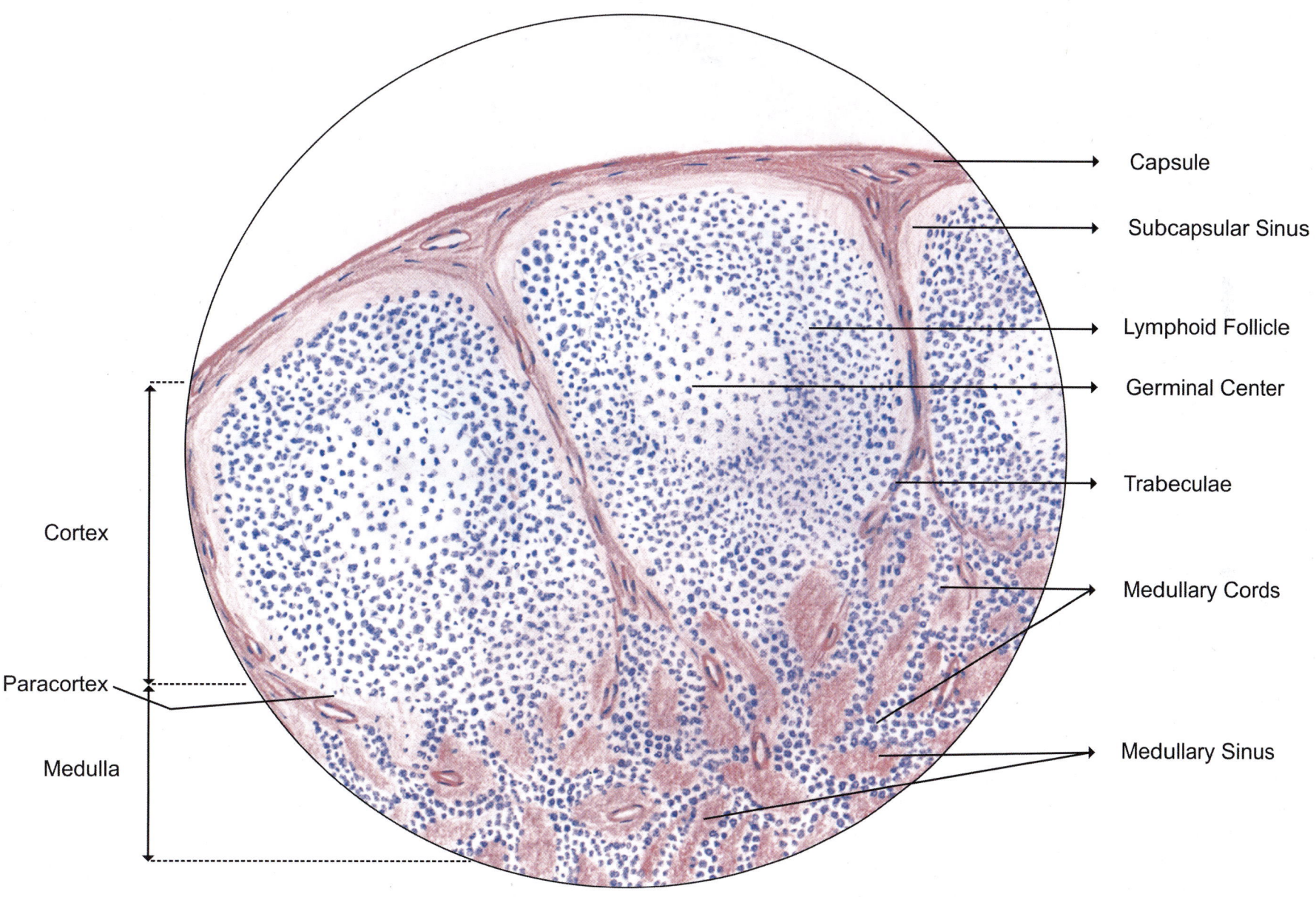

26. SPLEEN

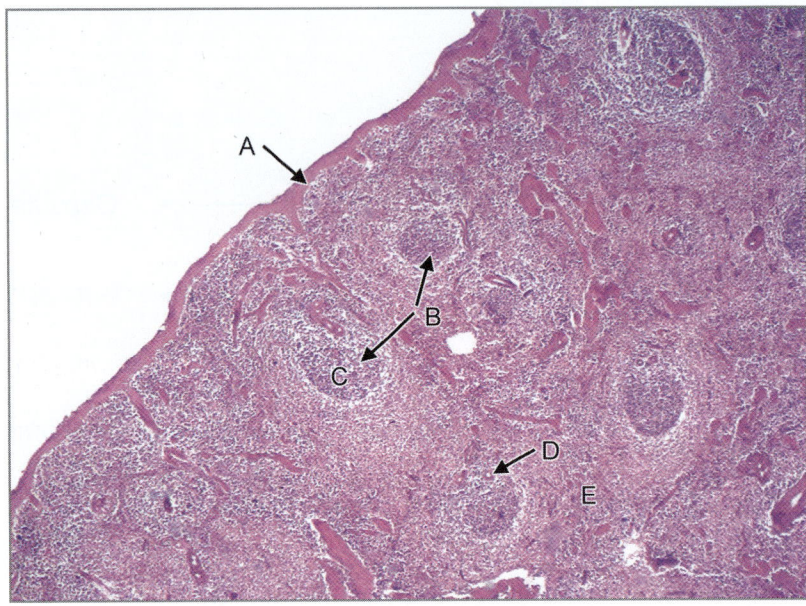

A	Capsule
B	White Pulp
C	Germinal Center
D	Eccentrically Placed Central Artery
E	Red Pulp

Identification Points

1. **Red pulp, white pulp differentiated.**
2. **White pulp—lymphoid aggregations with eccentric central artery.**
3. **Red pulp contains splenic cords surrounded by sinusoids.**

- Spleen has thick capsule, sends septa into substance of spleen.
- White pulp is aggregation of lymphocytes around the artery—periarterial lymphatic sheath (PALS) made of T lymphocytes. At some places it forms lymphatic nodules with germinal centers called as Malpighian bodies. They contain B lymphocytes.
- Red pulp forms the major part of spleen. It is made of lymphocytes arranged like branching and anastomosing cords along the sinusoids.
- Spleen is the largest hemolymphoid organ.
- Function—removes old red blood cells (RBCs), production of lymphocytes, removes blood-borne antigens. In fetal life it also acts as a site of erythrocyte production.
- Splenic circulation:
  - Central artery from white pulp enters red pulp and divides into straight vessels called as penicilli. It is then surrounded by sheath of macrophages and is called as ellipsoid which has a narrow lumen. Further it dilates to form ampulla and blood enters sinusoids of red pulp by two ways.
  - In closed circulation theory blood directly enters into sinusoids from ampulla. In open circulation theory blood passes out of capillaries between the cords and then enters sinusoids.

26. SPLEEN

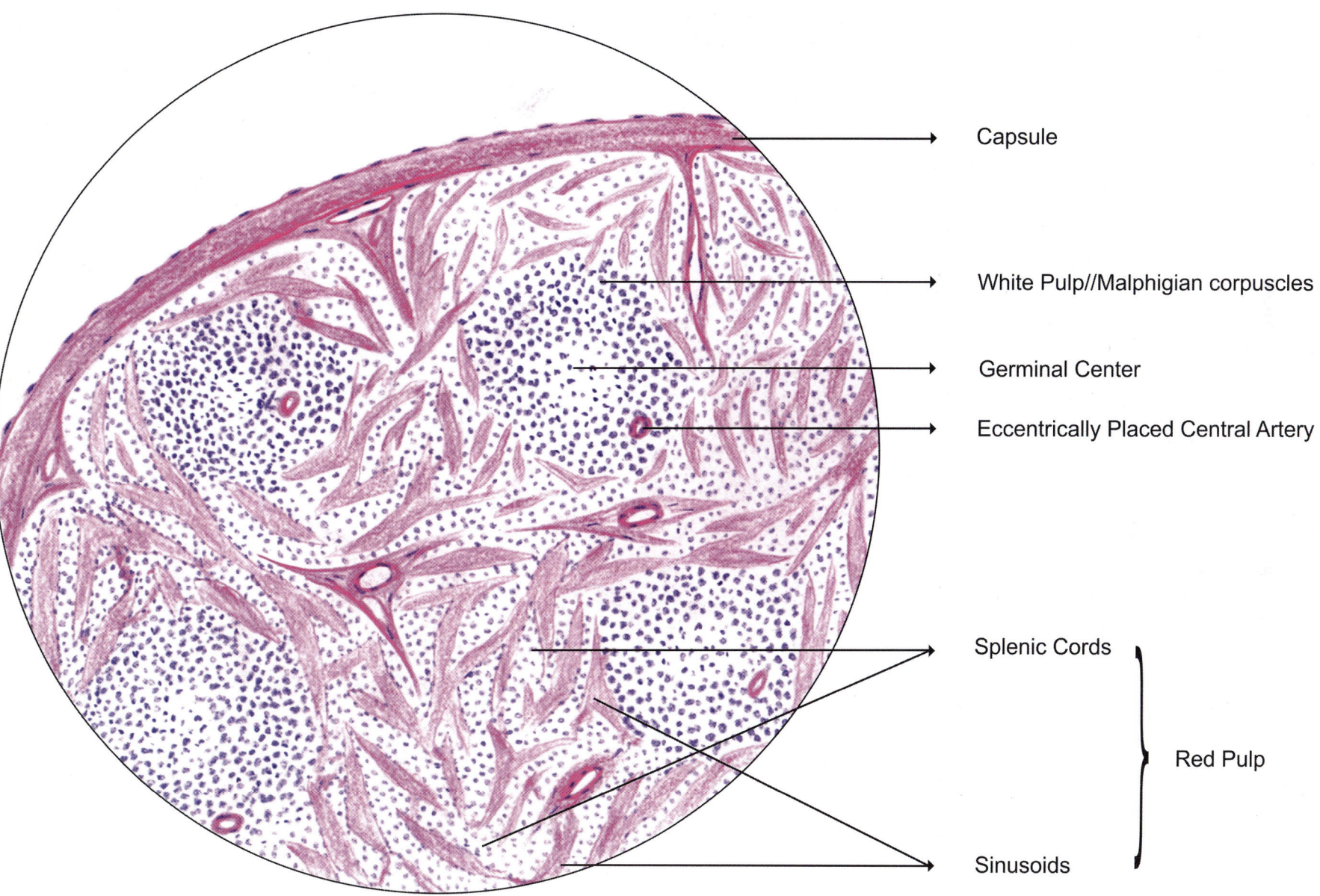

27. TONSIL

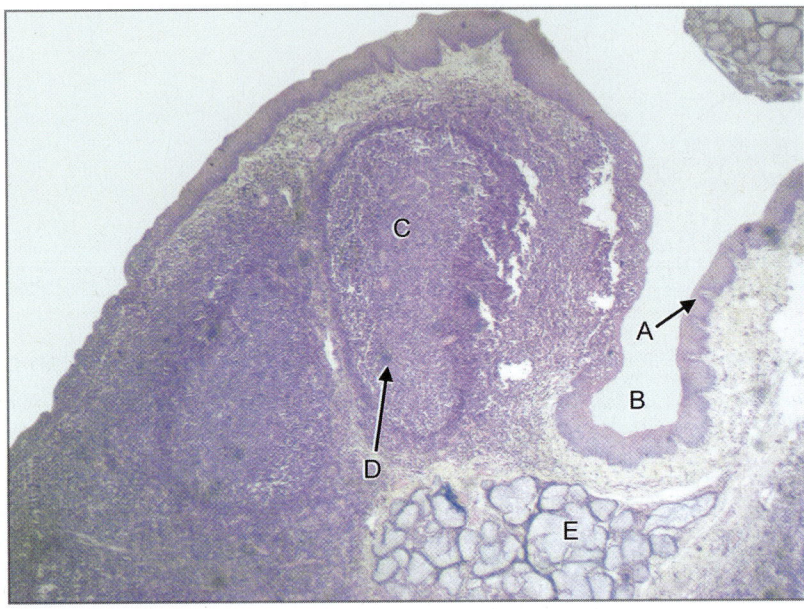

A	Stratified Squamous Non-keratinized Epithelium
B	Crypt
C	Lymphoid Follicle
D	Germinal Center
E	Mucus Acini

Identification Points

1. **Surface lined by stratified squamous non-keratinized epithelium.**
2. **Surface shows depressions called tonsillar crypts.**
3. **Lymphoid follicles with germinal center seen along the crypts.**

- Palatine tonsil is situated in tonsillar fossa, on lateral wall of oropharynx.
- It forms one of the constituents of Waldeyer's ring.
- It belongs to MALT (mucosa-associated lymphoid tissue). It is active during early life.
- Mucosal lining is non-keratinized stratified sqamous epithelium.
- Mucosal lining invaginate to form crypt which are characteristic of palatine tonsil.
- Lymphocytes aggregated in the form of follicles with a central germinal center along the crypts. Follicles mainly contain B lymphocytes. T lymphocytes lie outside the follicle.
- Mucus acini are seen in the deeper plane.

27. TONSIL

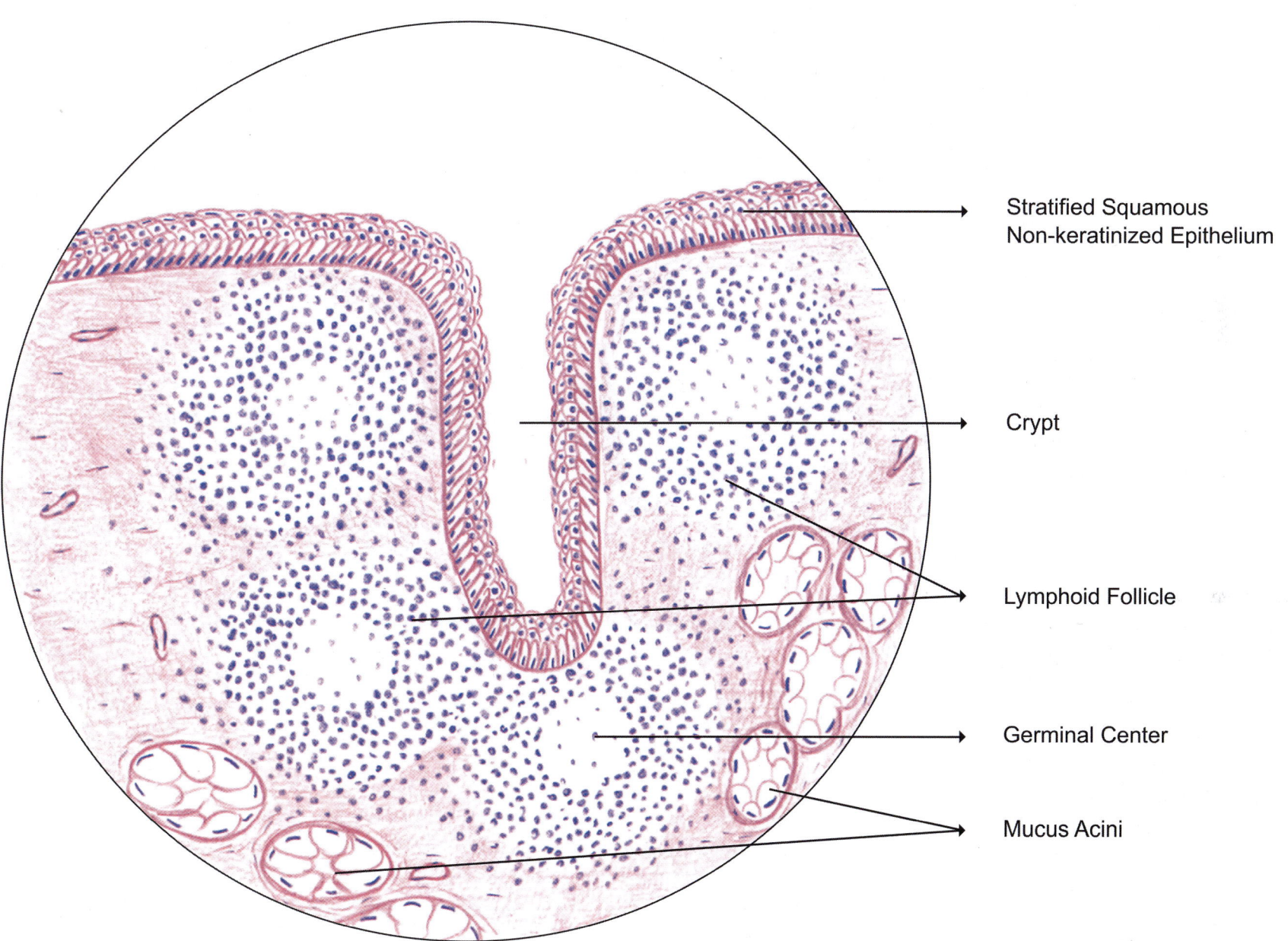

28. THYMUS

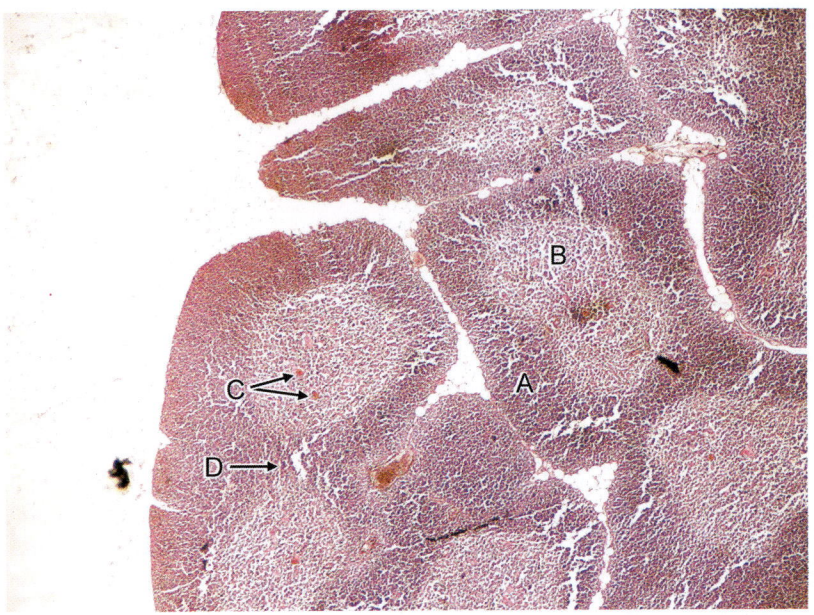

A	Cortex
B	Medulla
C	Hassall's Corpuscles
D	Incomplete Septa

Identification Points

1. **Lobules separated by incomplete fibrous septa.**
2. **Each lobule contains peripheral cortex of densely packed small lymphocytes and central medulla with sparsely arranged larger lymphocytes and Hassall's corpuscles.**

- Thymus is a primary lymphoid organ. It grows in size up to puberty and regress during adulthood.
- Capsule sends incomplete septa into the parenchyma, dividing it into lobules.
- Each lobule contains outer cortex and central medulla.
- Cortex is made of densely packed small lymphocytes.
- Also contains macrophages for phagocytosis of degenerating lymphocytes and epitheliocytes which provide supporting meshwork.
- Medulla of adjacent lobules are interconnected. It contains sparsely arranged larger lymphocytes and epitheliocytes.
- Degenerated epitheliocyte cell aggregations appear as concentric eosinophilic mass called Hassall's corpuscles in the medulla.
- Epithelioid cells form reticular system of thymus and forms blood-thymus barrier. Also produce hormones for proliferation and maturation of T lymphocytes.
- Function of thymus—differentiation of T lymphocytes.

28. THYMUS

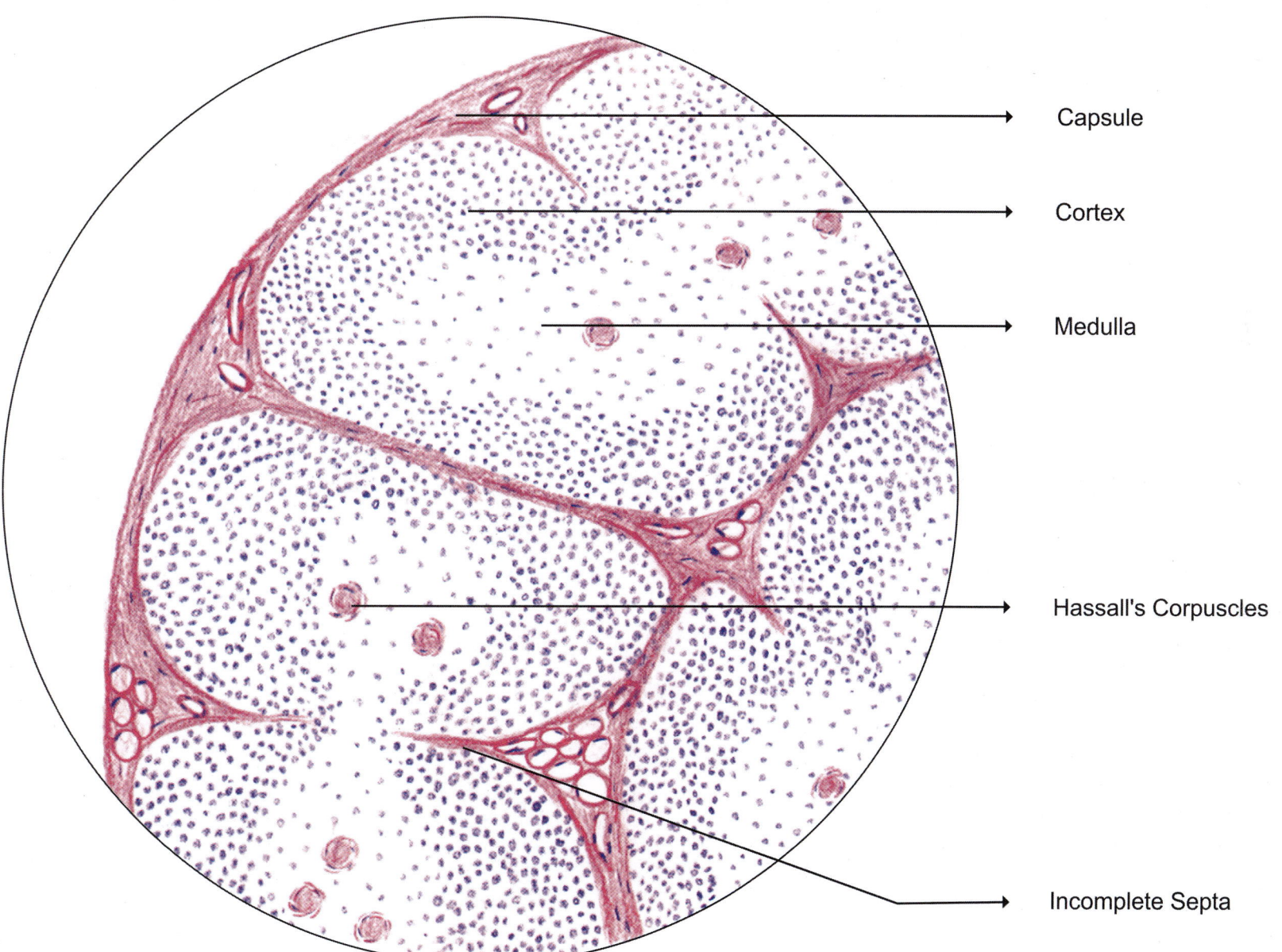

29. SEROUS SALIVARY GLAND

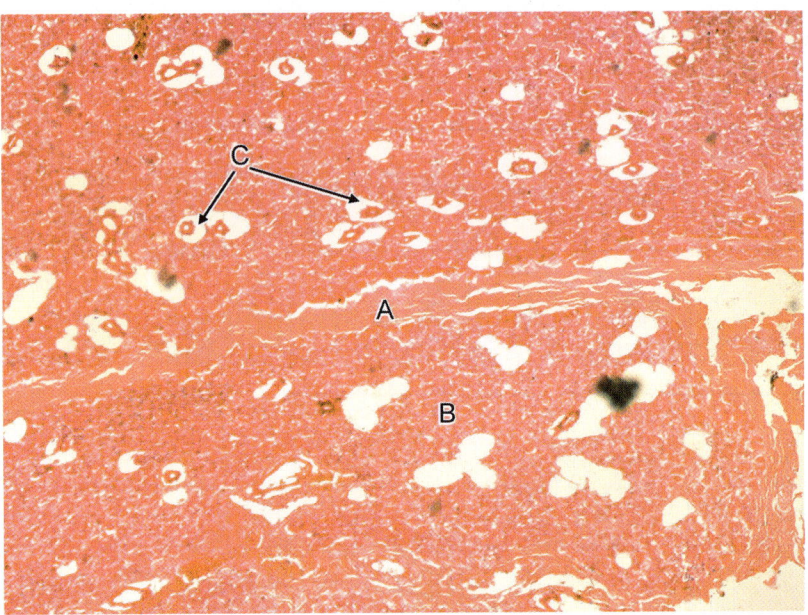

A	Connective Tissue Septum
B	Serous Acini
C	Intercalated Duct

Identification Points

1. **Serous acini with biphasic staining of pyramidal cells.**
2. **Striated and interlobular ducts are seen.**

- Capsular connective tissue sends septa, which divides gland into lobes and lobules.
- Each lobule contains secretory end pieces (acini) draining into intralobular then interlobular ducts.
- Serous acinus—small with narrow lumen, lined by pyramidal cells with round basal nucleus. Shows biphasic stain with H&E—apical part contains zymogen granules which stain eosinophilic, basal part takes basophilic stain.
- Intralobular ducts are of two types—intercalated duct and striated duct.
  – Intercalated duct lined by cuboidal cells.
  – Striated duct lined by columnar cells with basal infoldings of cell membrane giving it a striated appearance.
- These ducts help in transport of saliva and also modify the electrolyte content by adding potassium and bicarbonates and removing sodium ions. Also secrete immunoglobulin A (IgA).
- Interlobular ducts lined by stratified columnar cells, are seen within interlobular connective tissue.
- Contractile myoepithelial cells surround the secretory acini and help in release of secretions.

Example: Parotid salivary gland.

29. SEROUS SALIVARY GLAND

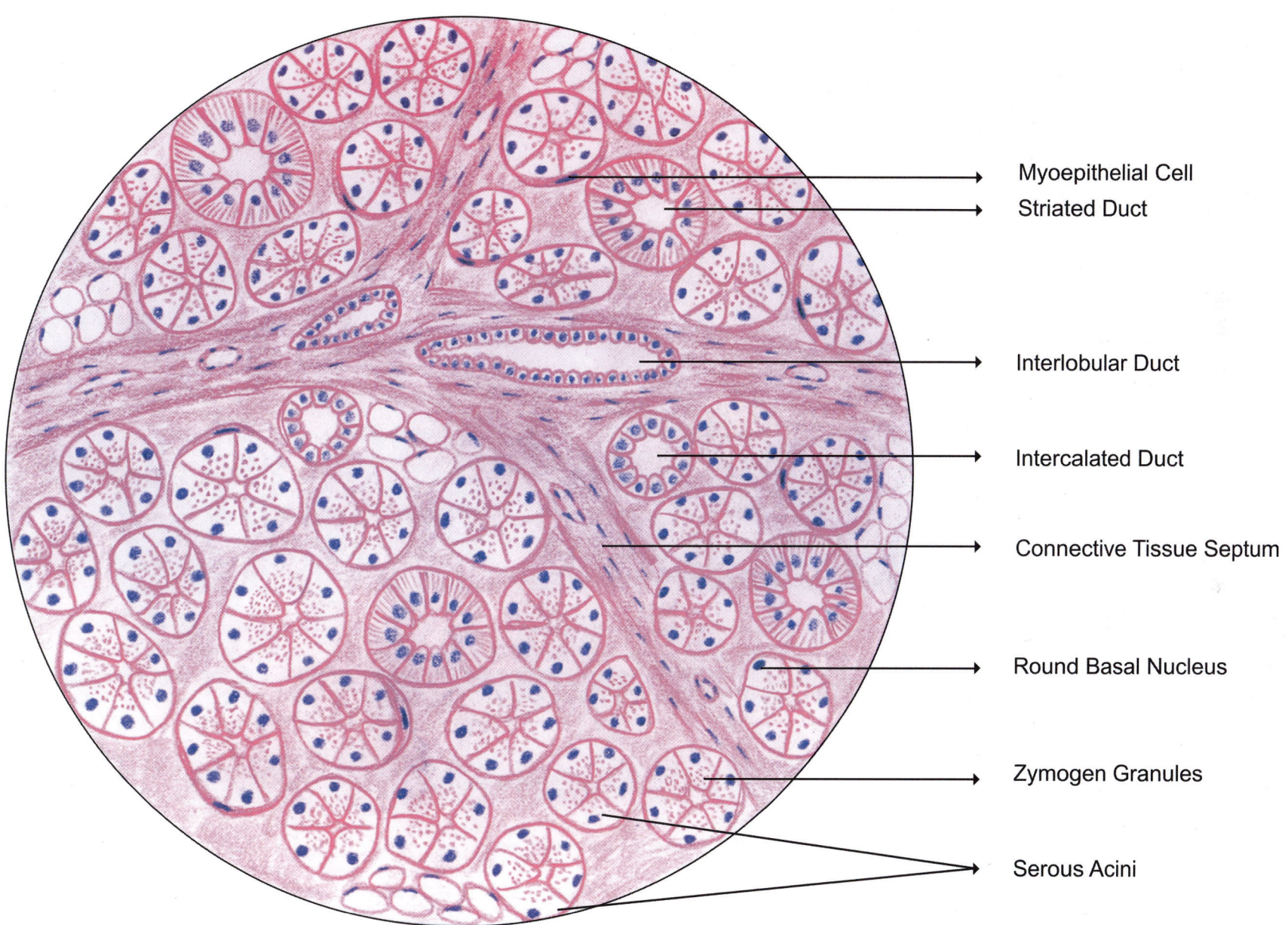

30. MUCUS SALIVARY GLAND

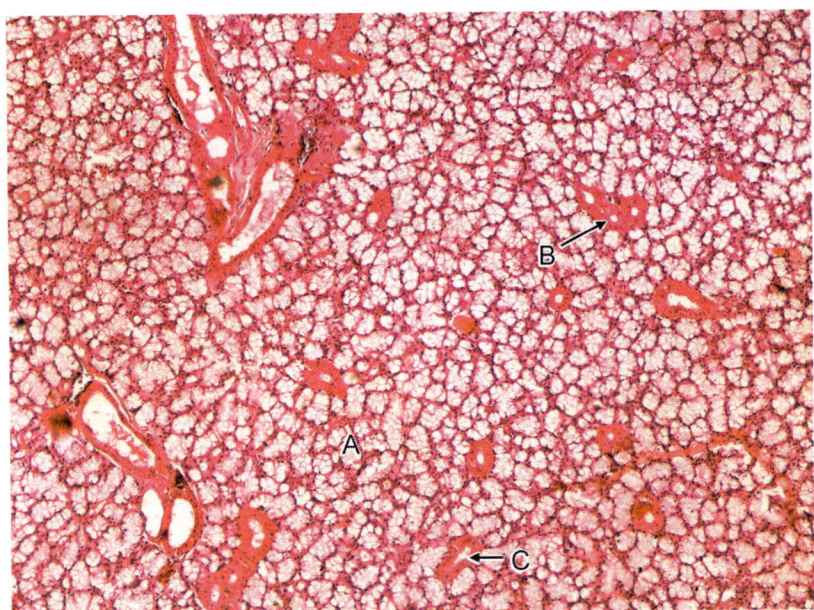

A	Mucus Acini
B	Intercalated Duct
C	Striated Duct

Identification Points

1. **Empty looking larger mucus acini with flattened basal nuclei and large lumen.**
2. **Interlobular ducts are seen.**

- Capsular connective tissue sends septa, which divides gland into lobes and lobules.
- Each lobule contains secretory end pieces (acini) draining into intralobular then interlobular ducts.
- Mucus acini are larger than serous acini with large lumen.
- Lined by columnar cells with flattened basal nuclei.
- Apical part of cells filled with pale-staining mucus droplets. As mucus does not take stain, cells look empty.
- Intralobular ducts present lined by cuboidal cells.
- Interlobular ducts lined by stratified columnar cells, are seen within interlobular connective tissue.
- Contractile myoepithelial cells surround the secretory acini and help in release of secretions.

Example: Sublingual salivary gland.

30. MUCUS SALIVARY GLAND

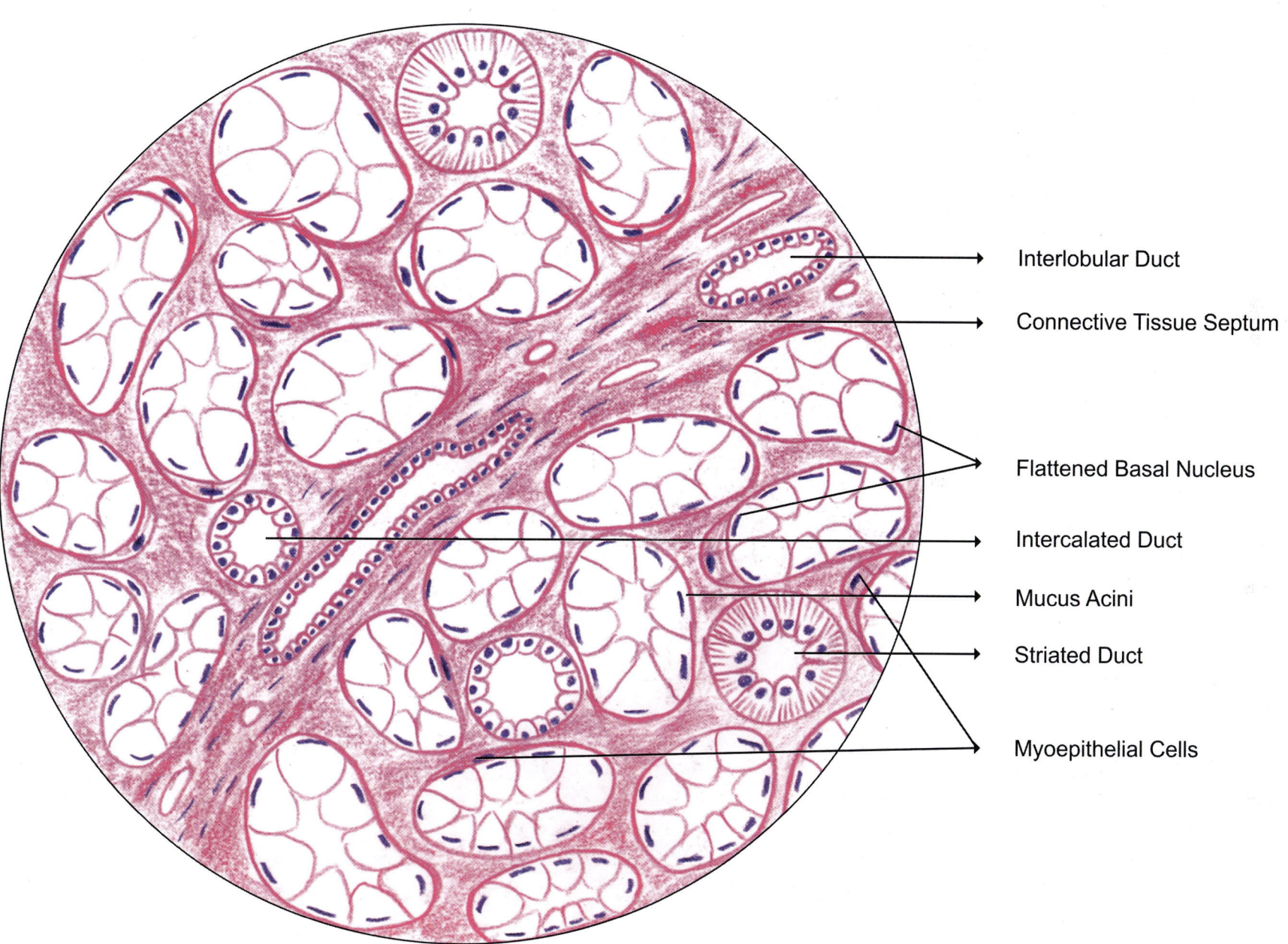

31. MIXED SALIVARY GLAND

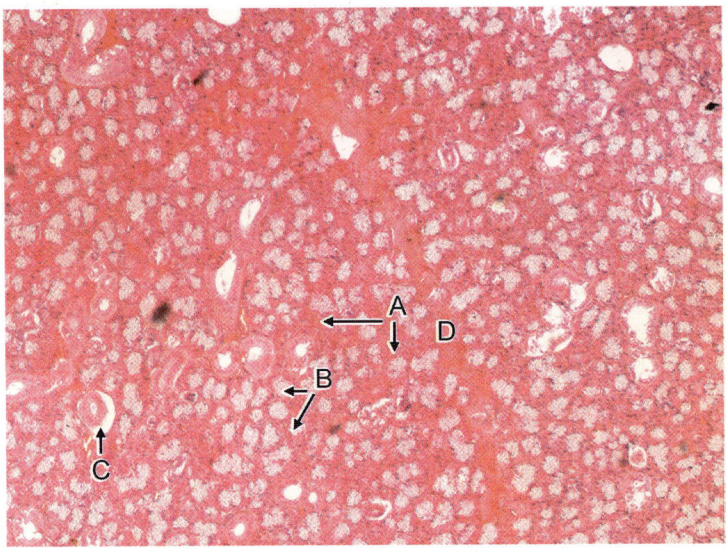

A	Serous Acini
B	Mucus Acini
C	Intercalated Duct
D	Connective Tissue Septum

Identification Points

1. Small serous acini with biphasic staining of pyramidal cells.
2. Empty looking larger mucus acini with flattened basal nuclei and large lumen.
3. Serous demilunes are seen capping the mucus acini.

- Capsular connective tissue sends septa, which divides gland into lobes and lobules. Each lobule contains secretory end pieces (acini) draining into intralobular then interlobular ducts.
- Serous acinus is small with narrow lumen, lined by pyramidal cells with round basal nucleus. Shows biphasic stain with H&E—apical part contains zymogen granules which stain eosinophilic, basal part takes basophilic stain.
- Mucus acini are larger than serous acini with large lumen, lined by columnar cells with flattened basal nuclei. Apical part of cells filled with pale-staining mucus droplets. As mucus does not take stain, cells looks empty.
- Serous demilunes seen—mucus acinus capped by serous cells.
- Intralobular ducts present lined by cuboidal cells.
- Interlobular ducts, lined by stratified columnar cells, are seen within interlobular connective tissue.
- Contractile myoepithelial cells surround the secretory acini and help in release of secretions.

Example: Submandibular salivary gland.

31. MIXED SALIVARY GLAND

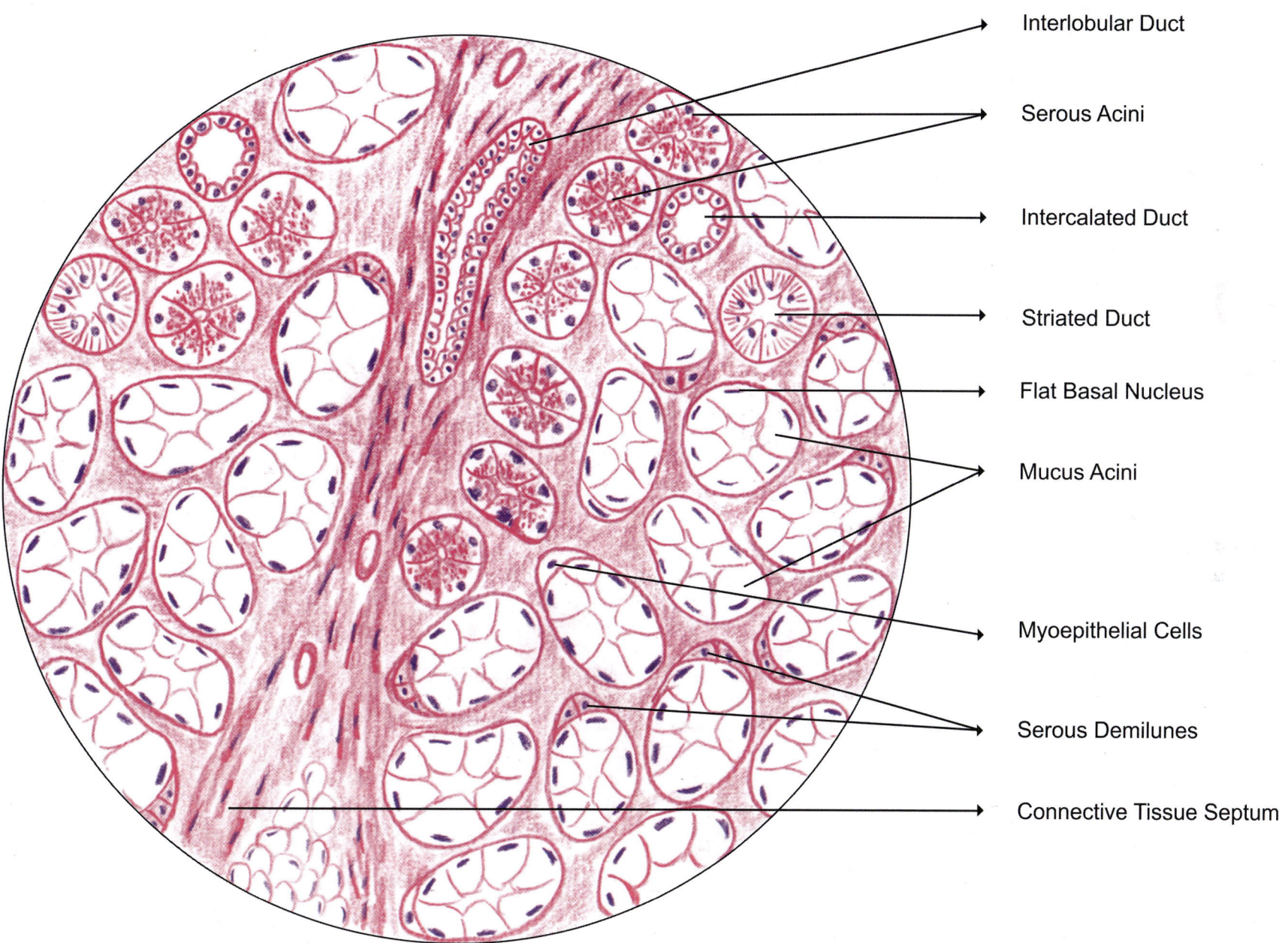

32. THICK SKIN

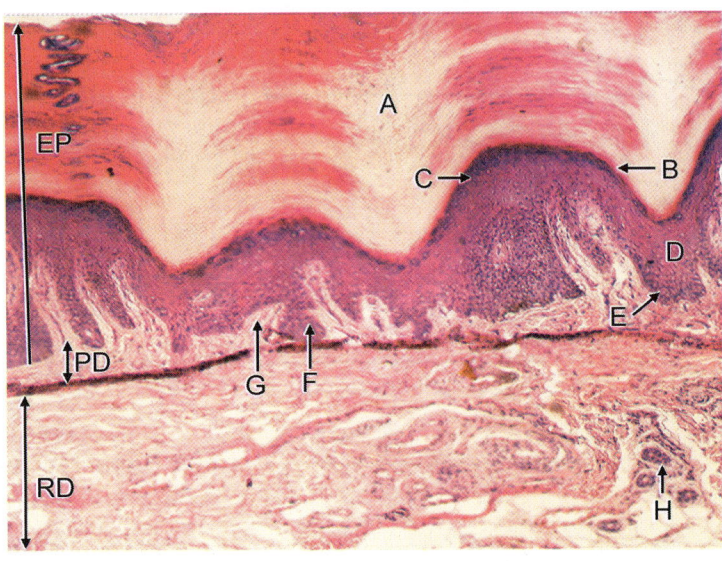

EP	Epidermis
PD	Papillary Dermis
RD	Reticular Dermis
H	Sweat Glands
E	Stratum Basale
D	Stratum Spinosum
C	Stratum Granulosum
B	Stratum Lucidum
A	Stratum Corneum
F	Epidermal Ridges
G	Dermal Papillae

Identification Points

1. **Outer epidermis—stratified squamous epithelium with thick keratin layer.**
2. **Inner dermis—connective tissue with sections of sweat glands and their ducts seen.**
3. **No hair follicles/sebaceous glands seen.**

Epidermis has five layers:

1. Stratum basale or stratum germinatum—is deepest where cell proliferation takes place, made of columnar cells.
2. Stratum spinosum/prickle cell layer—several layers of closely packed polyhedral cells joined by desmosomes.
3. Stratum granulosum—three to four layers of flattened cells containing keratohyalin granules.
4. Stratum lucidum—dead clear cells filled with keratin.
5. Stratum corneum—closely packed squames of keratin.

- Epidermis made up of two type of cells—keratinocytes and non-keratinocytes (melanocytes, Langerhans cells, Merkel cells).
- Dermis consists of papillary dermis and reticular dermis.
  - Papillary dermis is superficial, with loose connective tissue containing blood vessels and sensory nerve endings. It projects into the epidermis forming papillae.
  - Reticular dermis with dense connective tissue with bundles of collagen fibers.
- Skin appendages: Hair follicles, sebaceous gland, arrector pili muscle are absent.
  - Sweat gland is present.
- Thick skin found in palms and soles.

32. THICK SKIN

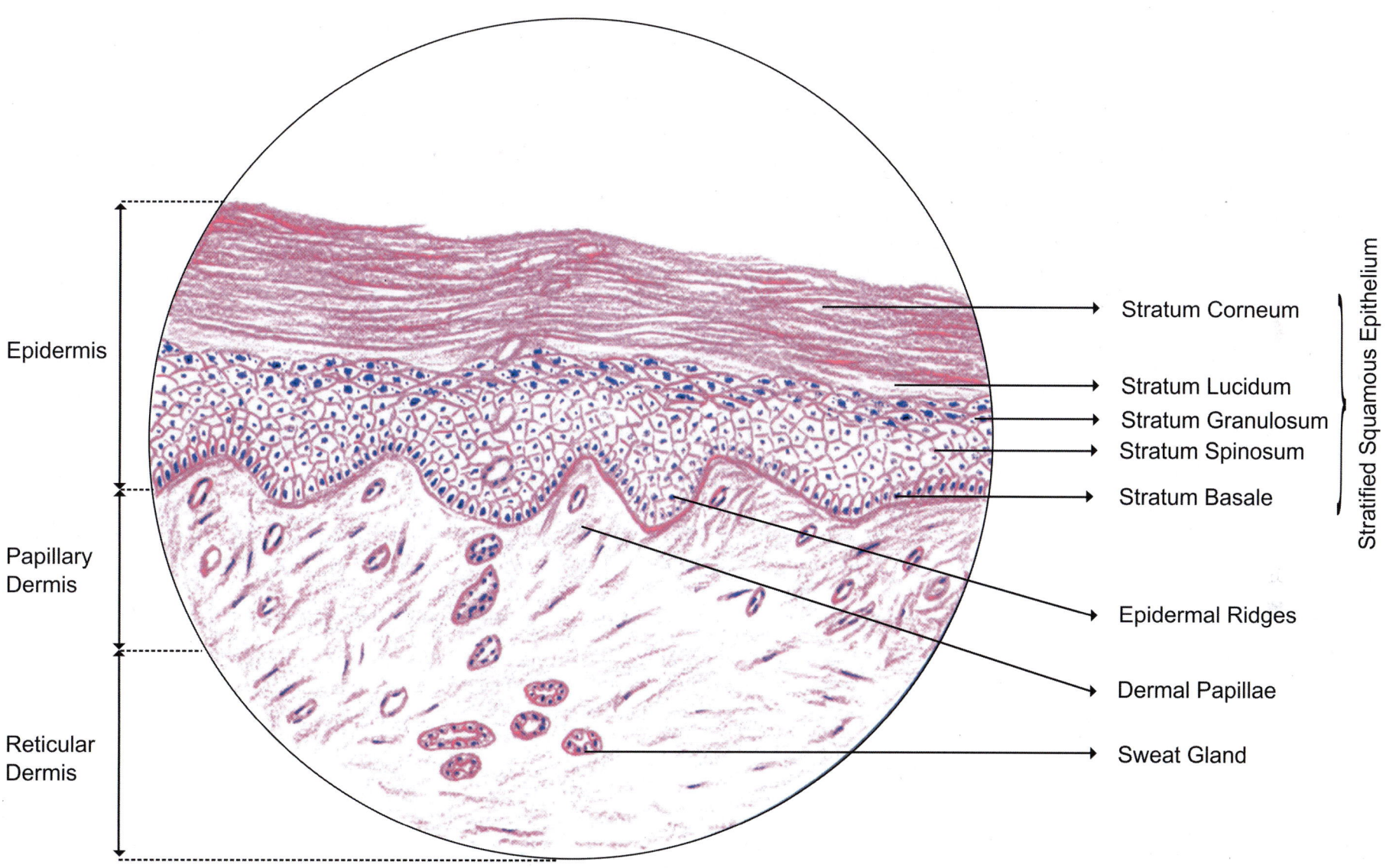

33. THIN SKIN

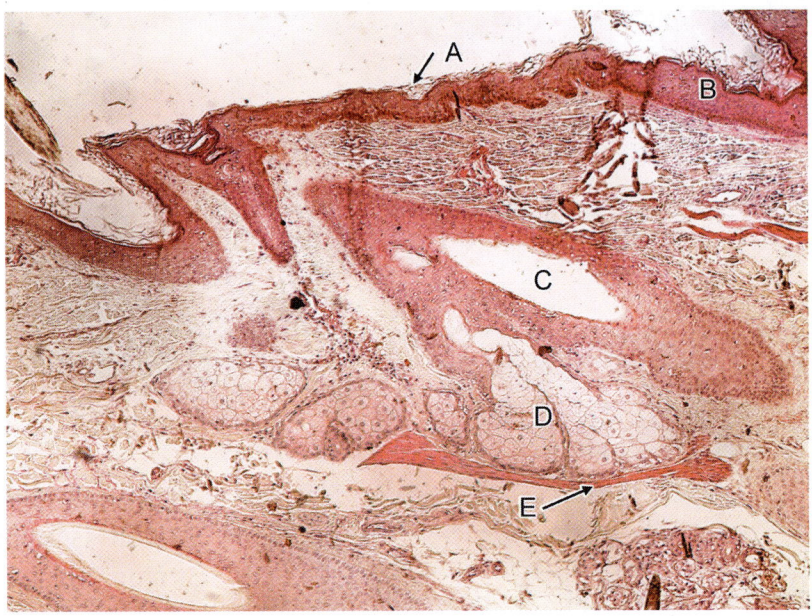

A	Keratin Layer
B	Epidermis
C	Hair Follicle
D	Sebaceous Gland
E	Arrector Pilorum Muscle

Identification Points

1. **Outer epidermis—stratified squamous epithelium with thin keratin layer.**
2. **Inner dermis—connective tissue with hair follicles, sebaceous glands, arrector pili muscle and sections of sweat glands seen.**

Epidermis has three layers:

1. Stratum basale or stratum germinatum—is deepest where cell proliferation takes place, made of columnar cells.
2. Stratum spinosum/prickle cell layer—several layers of closely packed polyhedral cells joined by desmosomes.
3. Stratum corneum—closely packed squames of keratin. Thinner than the thick skin.
- Epidermis made up of two type of cells—keratinocytes and non-keratinocytes (melanocytes, Langerhans cells, Merkel cells).
- Dermis consists of papillary dermis and reticular dermis.
  – Papillary dermis is superficial, with loose connective tissue containing blood vessels and sensory nerve endings. It projects into the epidermis forming papillae.
  – Reticular dermis with dense connective tissue with bundles of collagen fibers.

Skin Appendages

- Hair follicle—invagination of epidermis into dermis containing the cornified hair. Arranged obliquely at an angle to epidermis.
- Sebaceous gland —associated with hair follicle.
- Arrector pili muscle—bundle of smooth muscles which is arranged obliquely connecting the hair follicle with papillary dermis.
- Sweat glands and ducts seen.

33. THIN SKIN

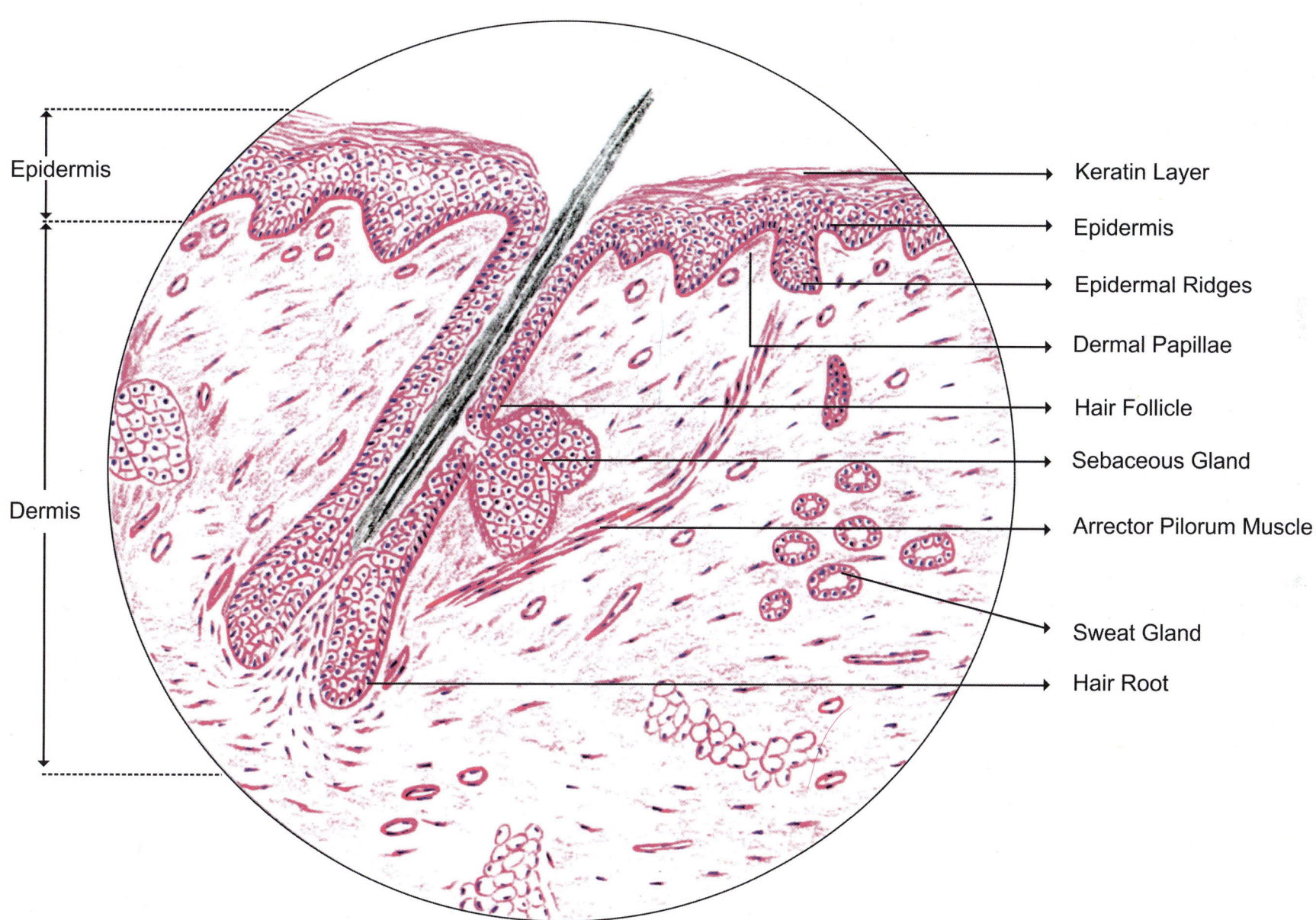

34. HAIR

Hair

It is derived from invagination of epidermis into dermis.

- Parts:
  1. Shaft—projects out from the body. Is a modification of stratum corneum.
     » Transverse section shows three layers from outside to inside:
        i. Cuticle—flattened overlapping keratinized cells.
        ii. Cortex—keratinized cuboidal cells and melanosomes.
        iii. Medulla—irregular-shaped large vacuolated cornified cells.
  2. Root—deep embedded part. Deep end of root is expanded to form the bulb.
     » It is invaginated from below by the vascular dermal papilla.
     » Root is surrounded by a tubular sheath called hair follicle.
- Hair follicle has two layers from inside out.
  - Inner root sheath- present only in the lower part, has three layers:
     i. Cuticle—inner most, flat cornified cells.
     ii. Huxley's layer—2 to 3 layers of cells with eosinophilic trichohyalin granules.
     iii. Henley's layer—single layer of keratinized cells.
  - Outer root sheath—continuous with stratum spinosum. A glassy membrane made of basal lamina separates it from dermis.
- Each follicle is divide into three segments:
  a. Infundibulum—from the surface of skin to opening of sebaceous ducts.
  b. Isthumus—from duct opening to arrector pili.
  c. Inferior segment—from the arrector pili to bulb.

34. HAIR

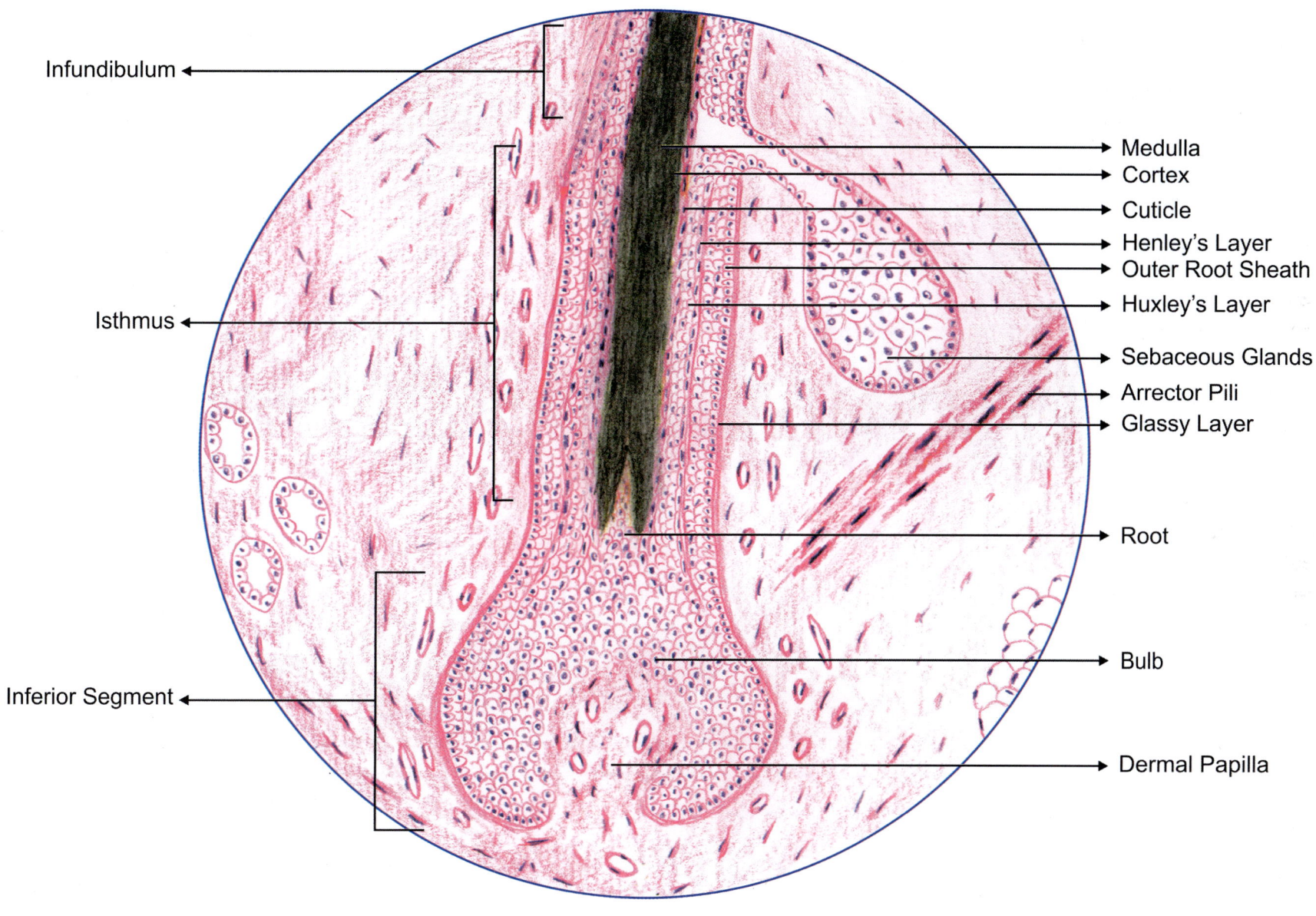

35. TRACHEA

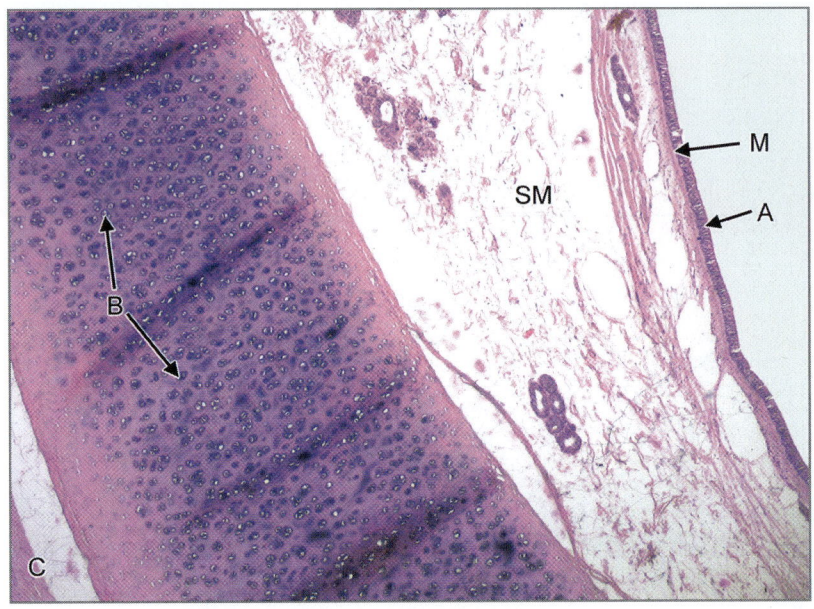

M	Mucosa
SM	Submucosa
H	Hyaline Cartilage Layer
A	Pseudostratified Ciliated Columnar Epithelium
B	Cell Nests of Hyaline Cartilage
C	Adventitia

Identification Points

1. Pseudostratified ciliated columnar epithelium with goblet cells lines the mucosa.
2. Serous and mucus glands in the submucosa seen.
3. Thick layer of hyaline cartilage present.

The trachea is formed of four layers:

1. **Mucosa**—lining epithelium is pseudostratified ciliated columnar epithelium with goblet cells. Lies over thin layer of connective tissue called lamina propria.
   - Cilia of pseudostratified ciliated columnar epithelium beat upward, so that mucus with trapped foreign particles are expelled.
   - Goblet cells and glands of submucosa secret mucus which traps dust particles.
2. **Submucosa**—Made of connective tissue with blood vessels and nerves.
   - Contains lot of serous and mucus glands. Elastic fibers are prominent.
3. **Cartilage**—C-shaped hyaline cartilage gives firm, flexible wall and contour to trachea.
   - Posterior ends of cartilage connected by trachealis muscle which completes the lumen and allows esophageal expansion.
4. **Adventitia**—made of connective tissue with blood vessels.

35. TRACHEA

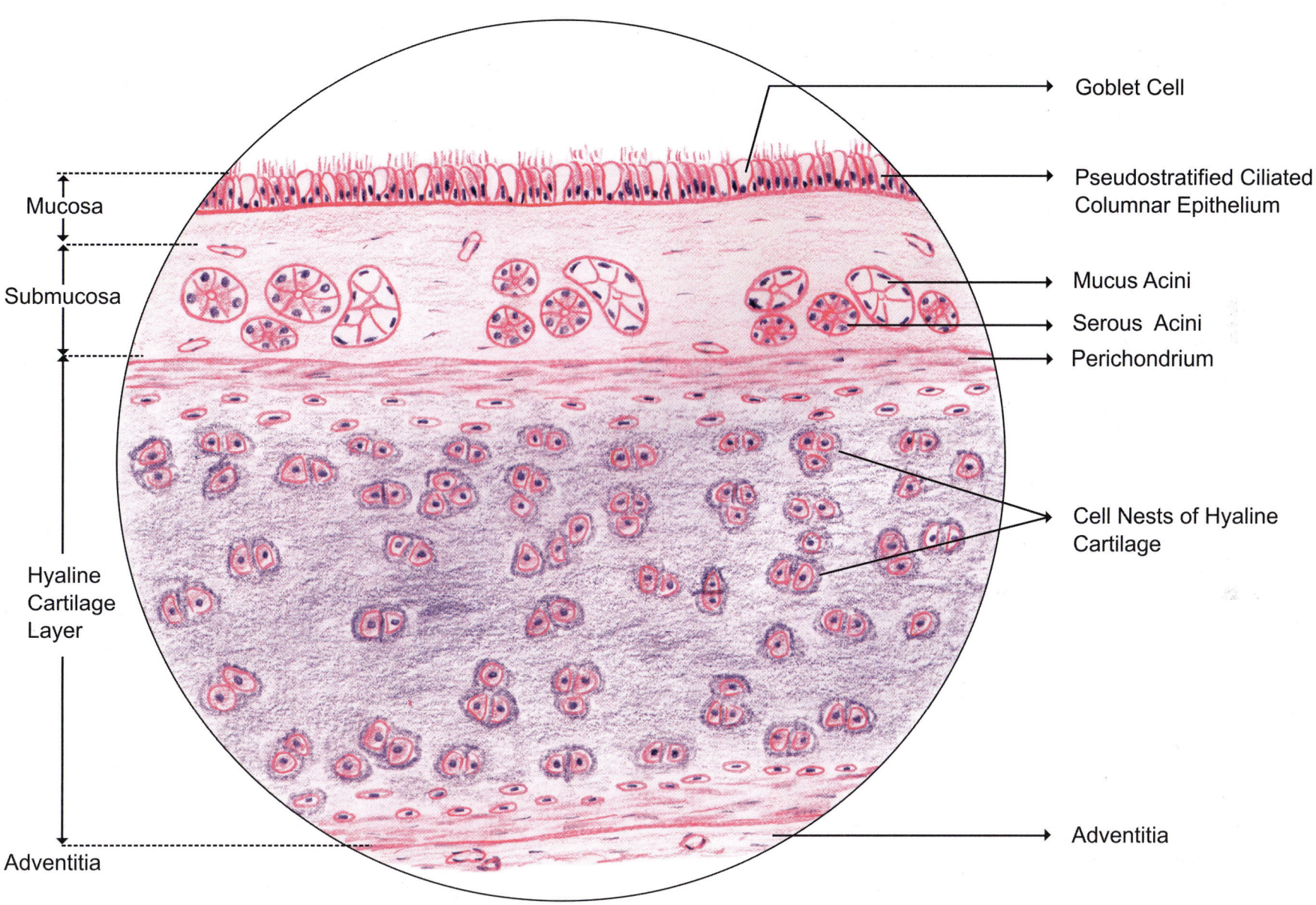

36. LUNG

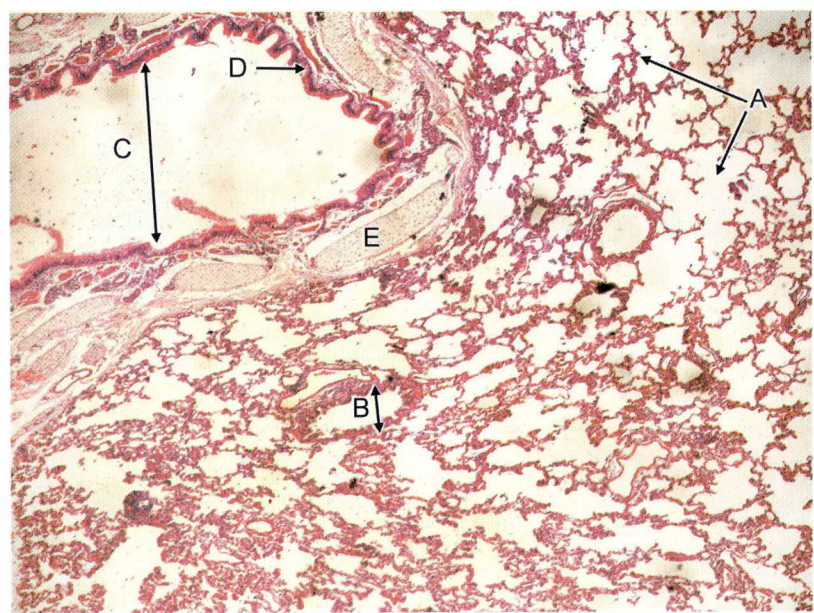

A	Alveoli
B	Bronchiole
C	Intrapulmonary Bronchus
D	Pseudostratified Ciliated Columnar Epithelium
E	Plates of Hyaline Cartilage

Identification Points

1. **Cut sections of intrapulmonary bronchi and bronchioles are seen.**
2. **Alveoli lined by simple squamous epithelium.**

- The respiratory tree consists of trachea, bronchi, bronchioles, terminal bronchioles, respiratory bronchioles and alveoli. Parts distal to respiratory bronchioles are involved in gas exchange.
- Thin-walled alveoli lined by flat cells. Two types of cells lines the alveoli:
  - Type I pneumocytes—simple squamous cells
  - Type II pneumocytes—surfactant producing.
- Lumen also contains macrophages called as dust cells which phagocytose the dust particles.
- Bronchus lined by pseudostratified ciliated columnar epithelium with goblet cells.
- Irregular plates of hyaline cartilage present in the bronchial wall.
- Bronchioles are smaller in size, 1 mm or less.
- Lined by simple ciliated columnar epithelium without goblet cells. Hyaline cartilage is absent in the wall. Has more smooth muscles and are prone for spasm.
- Respiratory lining epithelium changes to simple columnar at terminal bronchioles, cuboidal at respiratory bronchioles and squamous epithelium at alveoli.
- Blood gas barrier is formed by alveolar simple squamous epithelium with its basement membrane and capillary endothelium with its basement membrane.

36. LUNG

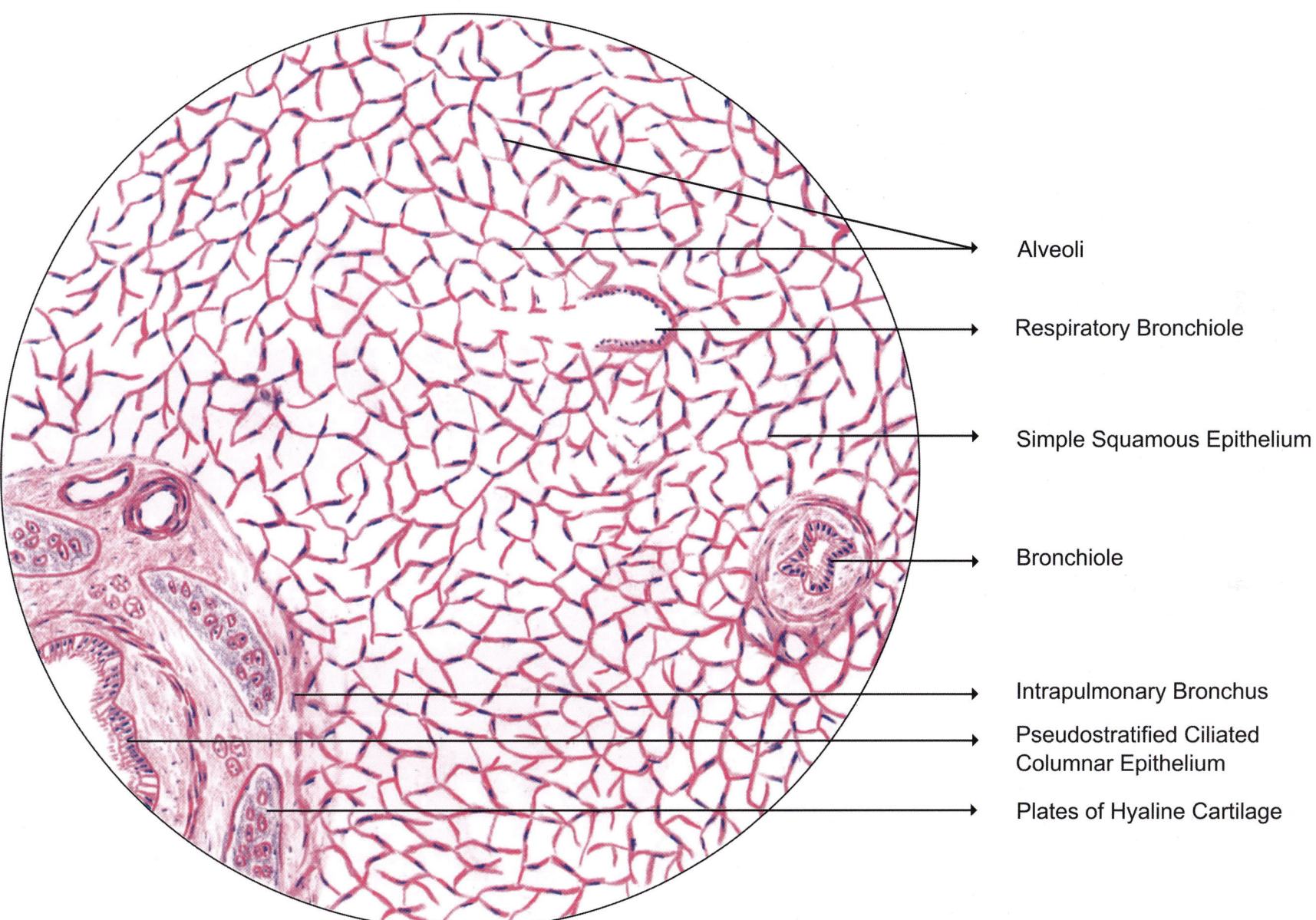

37. EPIGLOTTIS

Epiglottis

- It has a central core of elastic cartilage which gives support to the epiglottis.
- Outer surface covered by the mucous membrane:
  - Anterior surface (oral) and upper part of posterior surface (laryngeal) is lined by stratified squamous non-keratinized epithelium. Few taste buds are present.
  - Lower part of posterior surface (laryngeal) is lined by pseudostratified ciliated columnar epithelium.
- Submucosa contains connective tissue with mucous glands and few serous glands.

37. EPIGLOTTIS

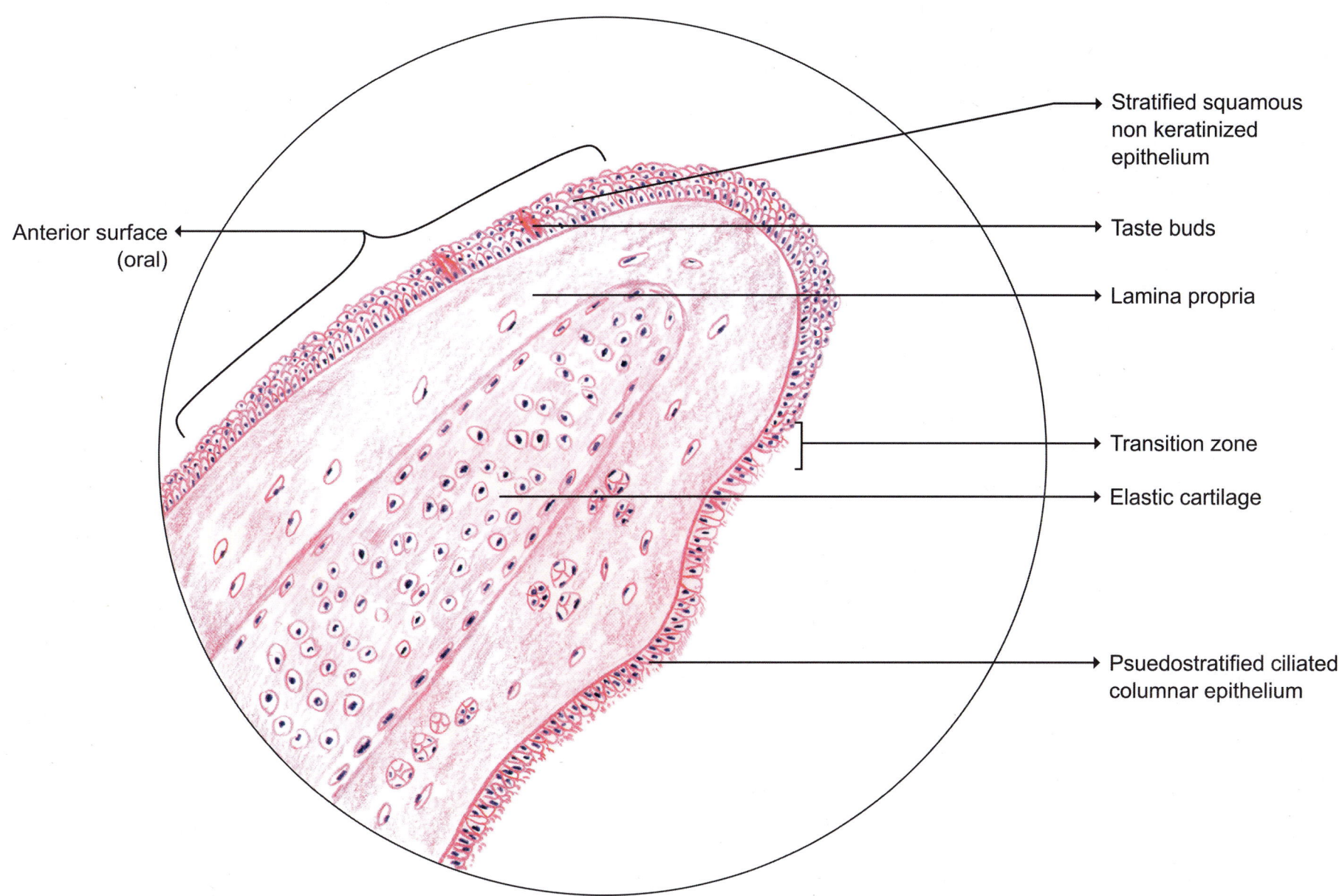

38. LIP

Lip

1. **External surface lined by thin skin and inner mucosal surface lined by oral epithelium.**
2. **Red margin—mucocutaneous junction of skin and mucous membrane.**
3. **Central core of skeletal muscle (orbicularis oris).**

- Skin—thin layered, made up of:
  - Epidermis—stratified squamous keratinized epithelium with hair follicle and sebaceous glands.
  - Dermis contains non-hair follicle associated sebaceous glands and sweat glands.
- Mucosa thick layered, lined by stratified squamous non-keratinized epithelium with prominent rete ridges.
- Beneath the mucosa, mucous secreting labial glands seen which helps to keep it moist.

38. LIP

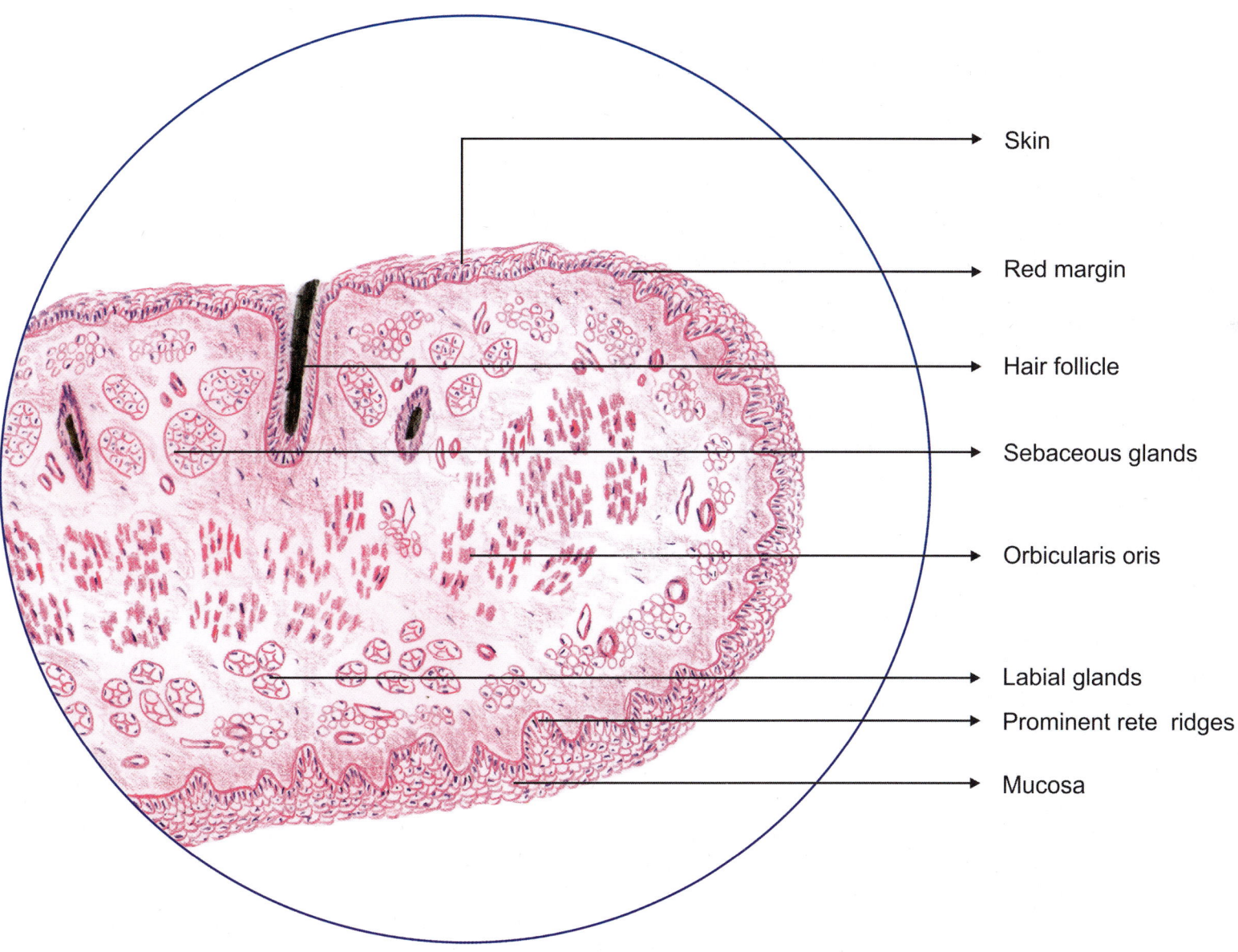

39(A). TONGUE: FILIFORM AND FUNGIFORM PAPILLAE

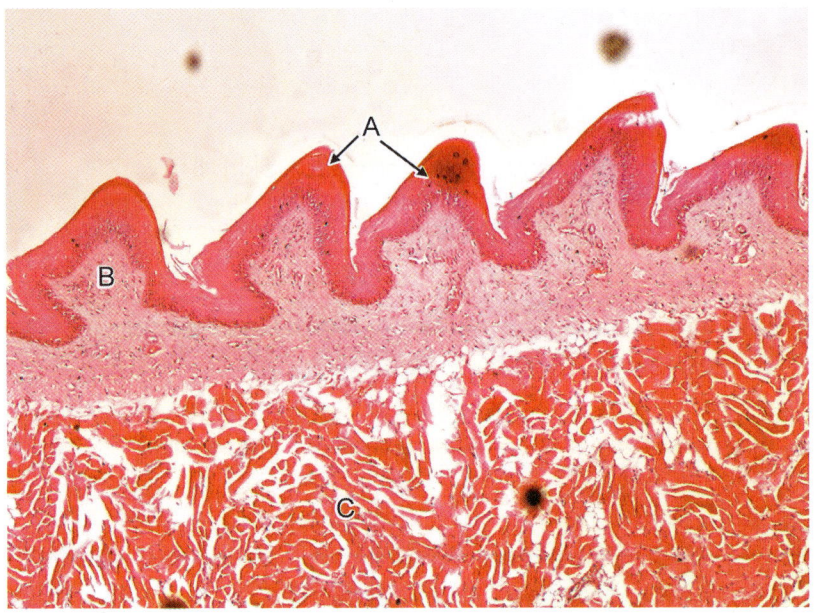

A	Stratified Squamous Non-keratinized Epithelium
B	Filiform Papillae
C	Skeletal Muscle

Identification Points

1. Surface lined by stratified squamous non-keratinized epithelium.
2. Surface shows projections called papillae.
3. Three types of papillae are—circumvallate/fungiform/filiform.
4. Circumvallate and fungiform papillae contain taste buds.
5. Cut sections of muscles and seromucous glands seen.

- Tongue is a muscular organ.
- Dorsal surface of tongue is lined by stratified squamous epithelium overlying the dense lamina propria with blood vessels, nerves and lingual glands.
- Surface is rough because of papillary projections.
- There are three types of papillae—filiform, fungiform and circumvallate papillae.
- Circumvallate papillae are only 8–12 in number and are situated in front of sulcus terminalis. They are large in size with base narrower than the apex. A circular sulcus surround the papillae, walls of which contain the taste buds. Bottom of the sulcus has the opening of serous glands.
- Fungiform papillae are scattered and round in shape with taste buds at the apical surface.
- Filiform are present in most of the area of dorsal surface, conical in shape. No taste buds. Mucosa covering these papillae are keratinized—makes the tongue surface rough.
- Taste buds are modified epithelial cells which are in contact with the nerves carry taste sensation. Tongue is richly innervated, taste is a special sensation.

39(A). TONGUE: FILIFORM AND FUNGIFORM PAPILLAE

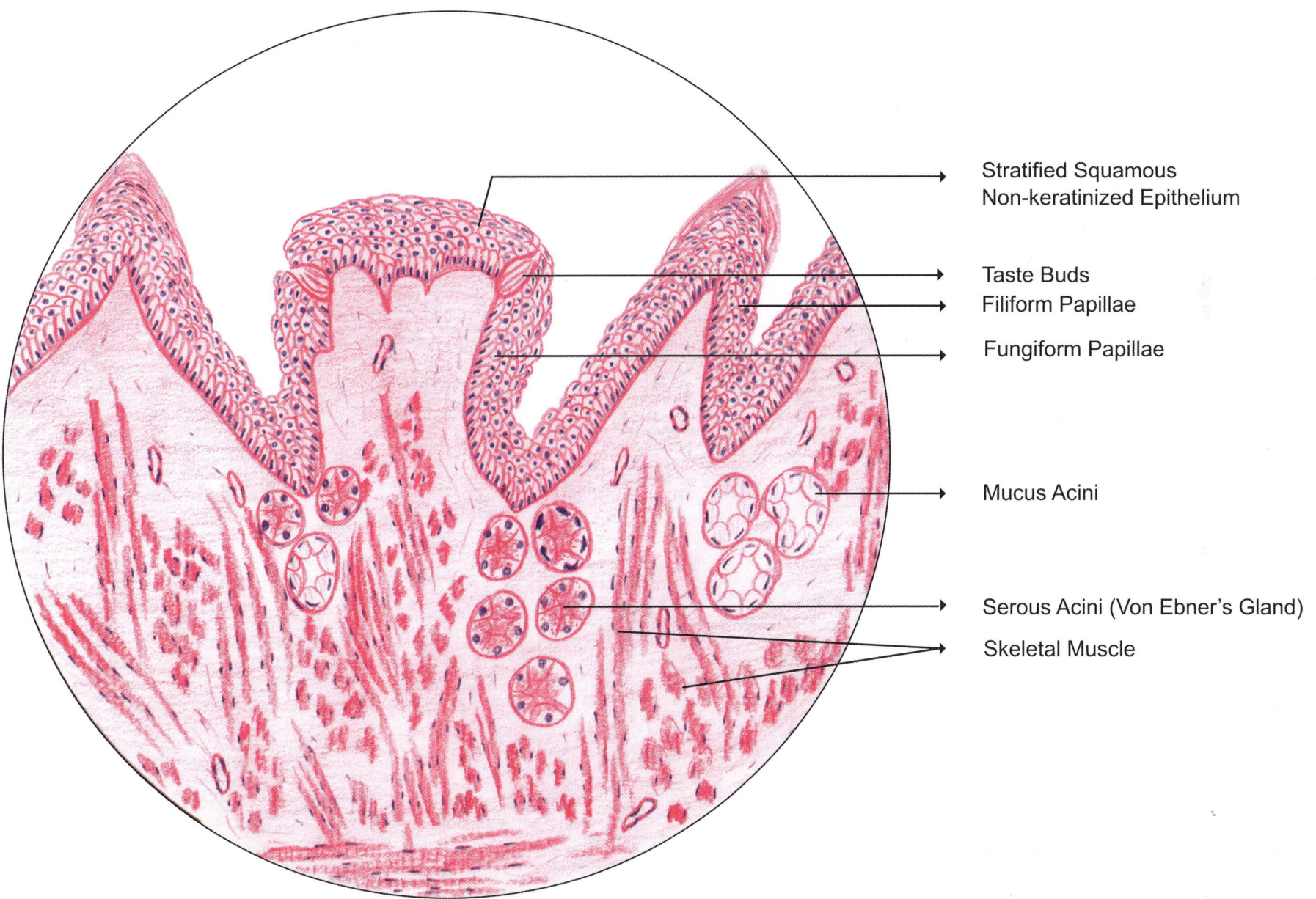

39(B). TONGUE: CIRCUMVALLATE PAPILLAE

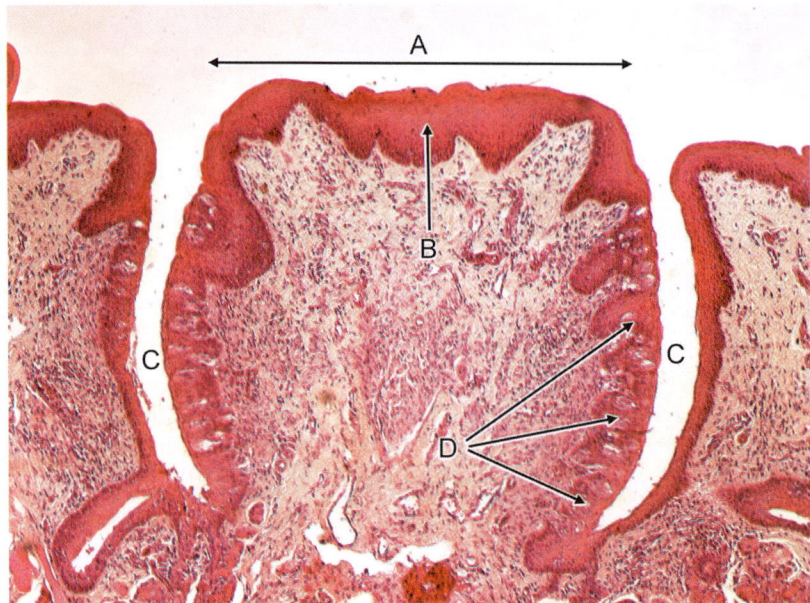

A	Circumvallate Papillae
B	Stratified Squamous Non-keratinized Epithelium
C	Circular Sulcus
D	Taste Buds

Identification Points

1. **Surface lined by stratified squamous non-keratinized epithelium.**
2. **Surface shows projection called papillae.**
3. **Three types of papillae are—circumvallate/fungiform/filiform.**
4. **Circumvallate and fungiform papillae contain taste buds.**
5. **Cut sections of muscles and seromucous glands seen.**

- Tongue is a muscular organ.
- Dorsal surface of tongue is lined by stratified squamous epithelium overlying the dense lamina propria with blood vessels, nerves and lingual glands.
- Surface is rough because of papillary projections.
- There are three types of papillae—filiform, fungiform and circumvallate papillae.
- Circumvallate papillae are only 8–12 in number and are situated in front of sulcus terminalis. They are large in size with base narrower than the apex. A circular sulcus surround the papillae, walls of which contain the taste buds. Bottom of the sulcus has the opening of serous glands.
- Taste buds are modified epithelial cells which are in contact with the nerves which carry taste sensation. Tongue is richly innervated, taste is a special sensation.

39(B). TONGUE: CIRCUMVALLATE PAPILLAE

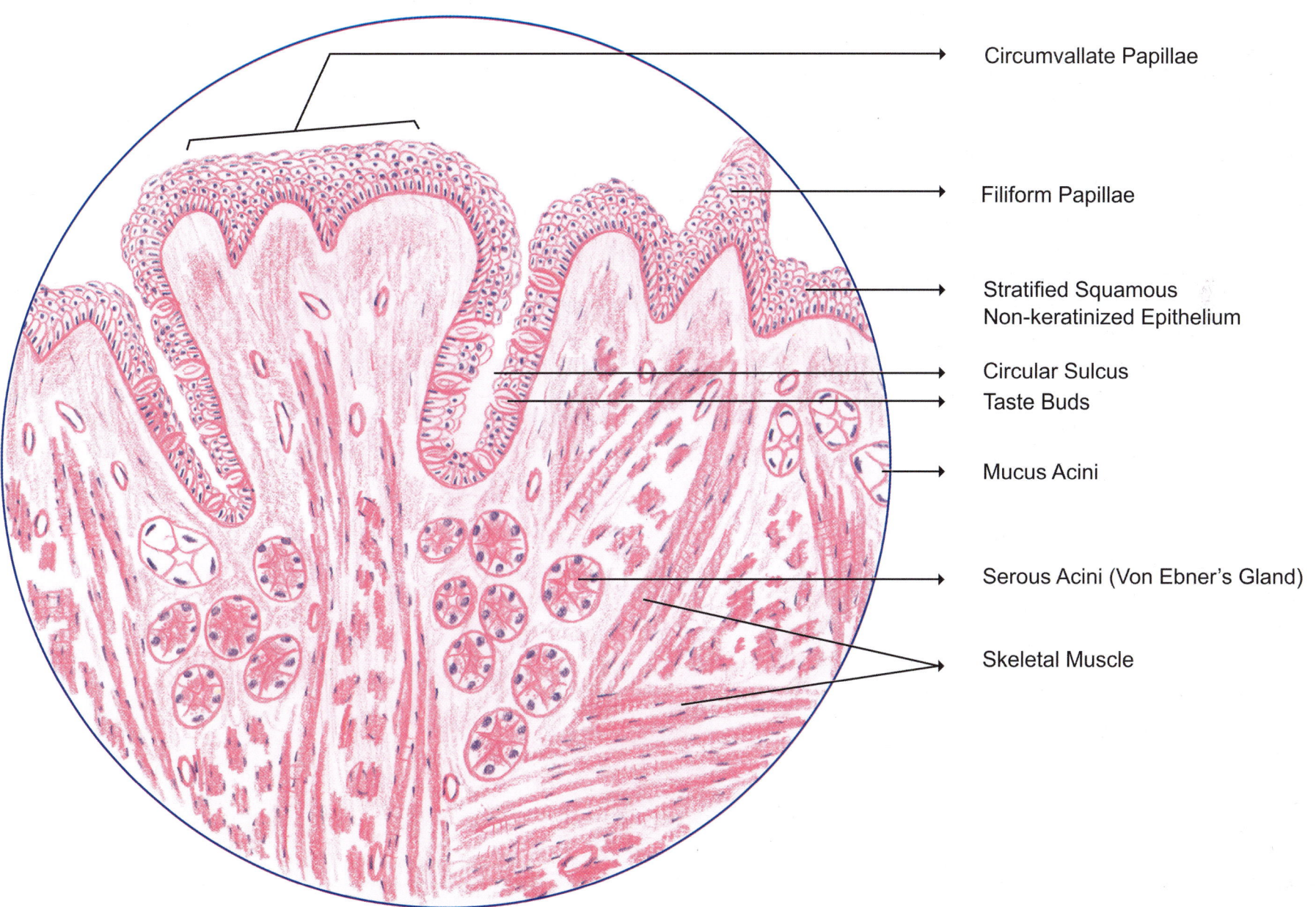

- Circumvallate Papillae
- Filiform Papillae
- Stratified Squamous Non-keratinized Epithelium
- Circular Sulcus
- Taste Buds
- Mucus Acini
- Serous Acini (Von Ebner's Gland)
- Skeletal Muscle

40. TOOTH

Tooth

Dried tooth—longitudinal section, non-decalcified and unstained.

Made of outer crown and inner embedded root

- Longitudinal section shows three layers:
1. **Enamel**—outer portion covering the dentin in region of crown.
   – Made of hydroxyapatite crystals of calcium phosphate and carbonate.
2. **Dentine**—middle part made of calcified gylcosaminoglycans and collagen fibers.
   – Permeated by fine canaliculi radiating from pulp cavity towards the enamel.
   – Over the root the dentin is covered by cementum which attaches to bony socket by periodontal ligament.
3. **Pulp**—innermost layer in the pulp cavity and root canal.
   – Contains gelatinous loose connective tissue with cells, collagen fiber, blood vessels, lymphatics and nerve fibers.

40. TOOTH

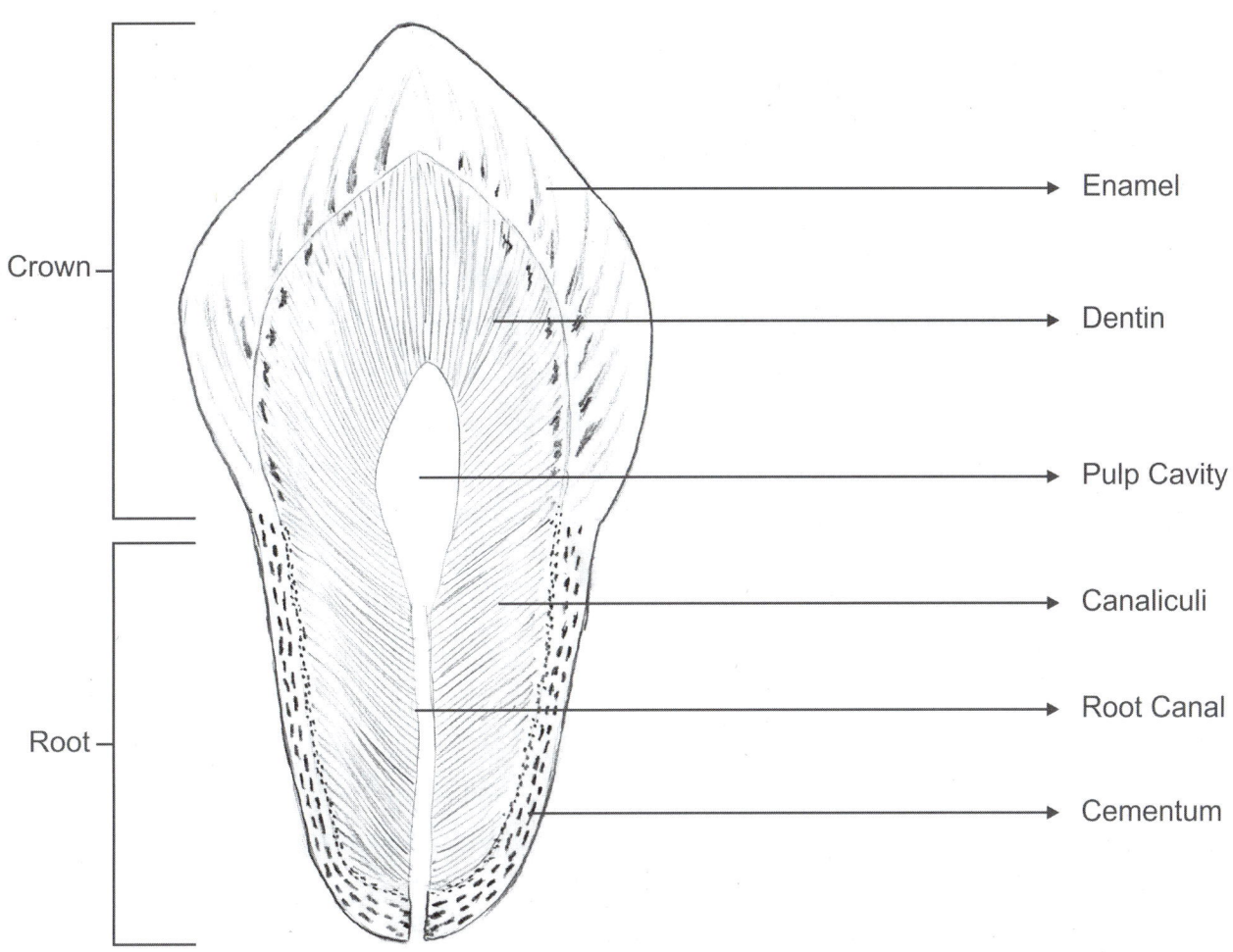

41. ESOPHAGUS

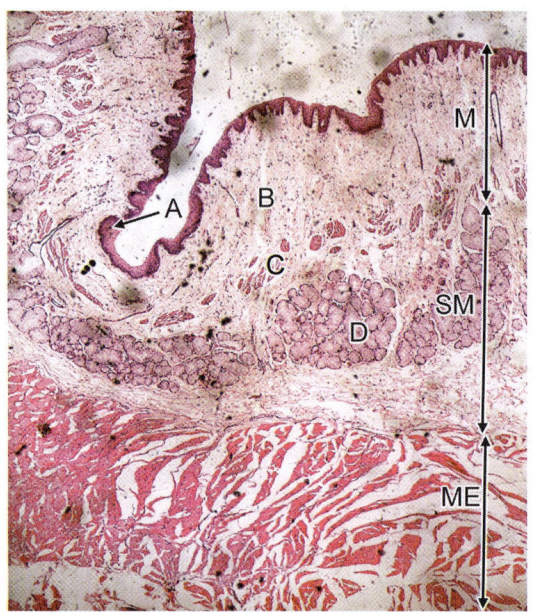

M	Mucosa
SM	Submucosa
ME	Muscularis Externa
B	Lamina Propria
C	Muscularis Mucosa
D	Esophageal Glands
A	Stratified Squamous Non-keratinized Epithelium

Identification Points

1. **Mucosa lined by non-keratinized stratified squamous epithelium.**
2. **Mucus secreting esophageal glands in the submucosal layer.**

- Normally esophagus lumen is collapsed with longitudinal mucosal folds. Functionally it is a passage for bolus of food.
- Four layers of gastrointestinal (GI) tract—mucosa, submucosa, muscularis externa, adventitia/serosa.
  1. Mucosa
     » Epithelium made of non-keratinized stratified squamous epithelium.
     » Lamina propria—loose connective tissue with blood vessels.
     » Muscularis mucosa is two layered—inner longitudinal, outer circular (smooth muscle).
  2. Submucosa—loose connective tissue with blood vessels and nerves. Also contains mucus secreting esophageal glands. The secretions from the glands help in lubrication of lumen and protect the mucosa.
  3. Muscularis externa—inner circular, outer longitudinal layer. Muscle fibers are skeletal muscle proximally, mixed in the middle portion and distally only smooth muscle.
  4. Adventitia/serosa—loose connective tissue called adventitia with blood vessels and nerves.

41. ESOPHAGUS

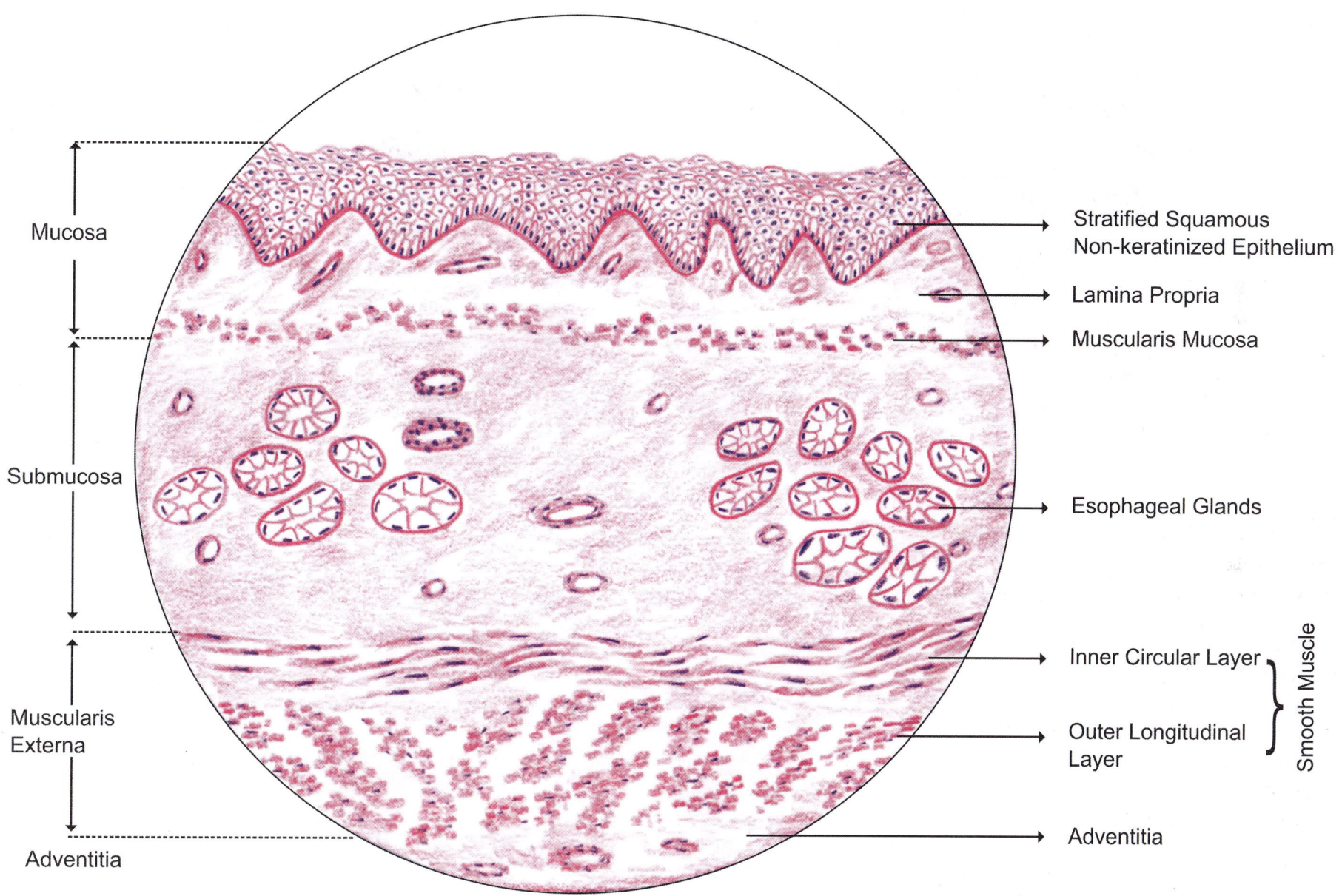

42. STOMACH: FUNDUS AND BODY

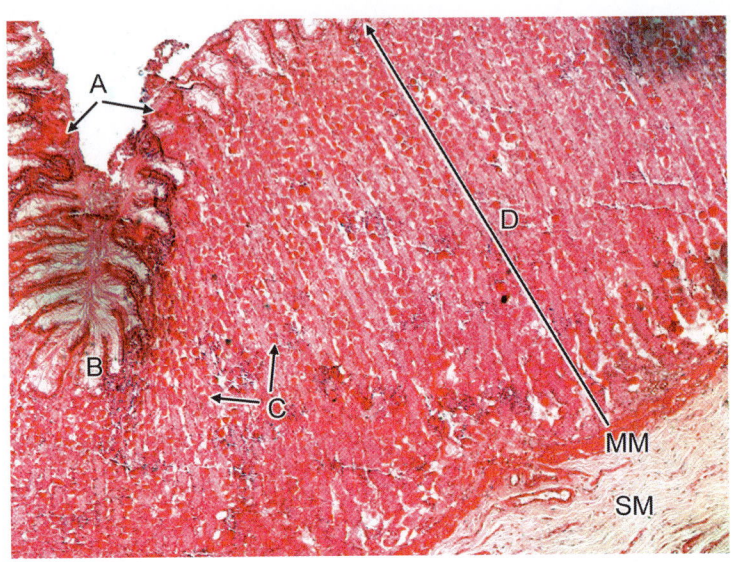

SM	Submucosa
MM	Muscularis Mucosa
A	Simple Columnar Epithelium
B	Gastric Pit
D	Gastric Glands
C	Parietal Cells

Identification Points

1. Mucosal lining is simple columnar epithelium.
2. Shallow gastric pits present.
3. Lamina propria filled with deep straight tubular glands with parietal and chief cells.

- Mucosal folds of stomach are called rugae, are temporary.
- It has four layers—mucosa, submucosa, muscularis externa, serosa.
    1. Mucosa
        » Lining epithelium is simple columnar type. Invagination of surface lining into the lamina propria is called gastric pit which is shallow. Depth of gastric pits is about one-third of thickness of mucosa.
        » Lamina propria filled with simple straight tubular gastric glands which open into bottom of the pits. Gastric glands lined by parietal cell, chief cell, mucus neck cells.
        » Muscularis mucosa—inner circular and outer longitudinal layer of smooth muscles.
    2. Submucosa—loose connective tissue with blood vessels and nerves.
    3. Muscularis externa (three layers)—inner oblique, middle circular, outer longitudinal smooth muscle.
    4. Serosa—membrane made of a simple squamous epithelium.
- Parietal cells also called oxyntic cells. They secrete gastric acid and intrinsic factor. Cells are large and eosinophilic; present in the upper part of the glands.
- Chief cells also called zymogen cells. They secrete pepsinogen. They are basophilic, present in the lower part of glands.
- Mucus neck cells—secrete mucus which helps in protection of mucosa.

42. STOMACH: FUNDUS AND BODY

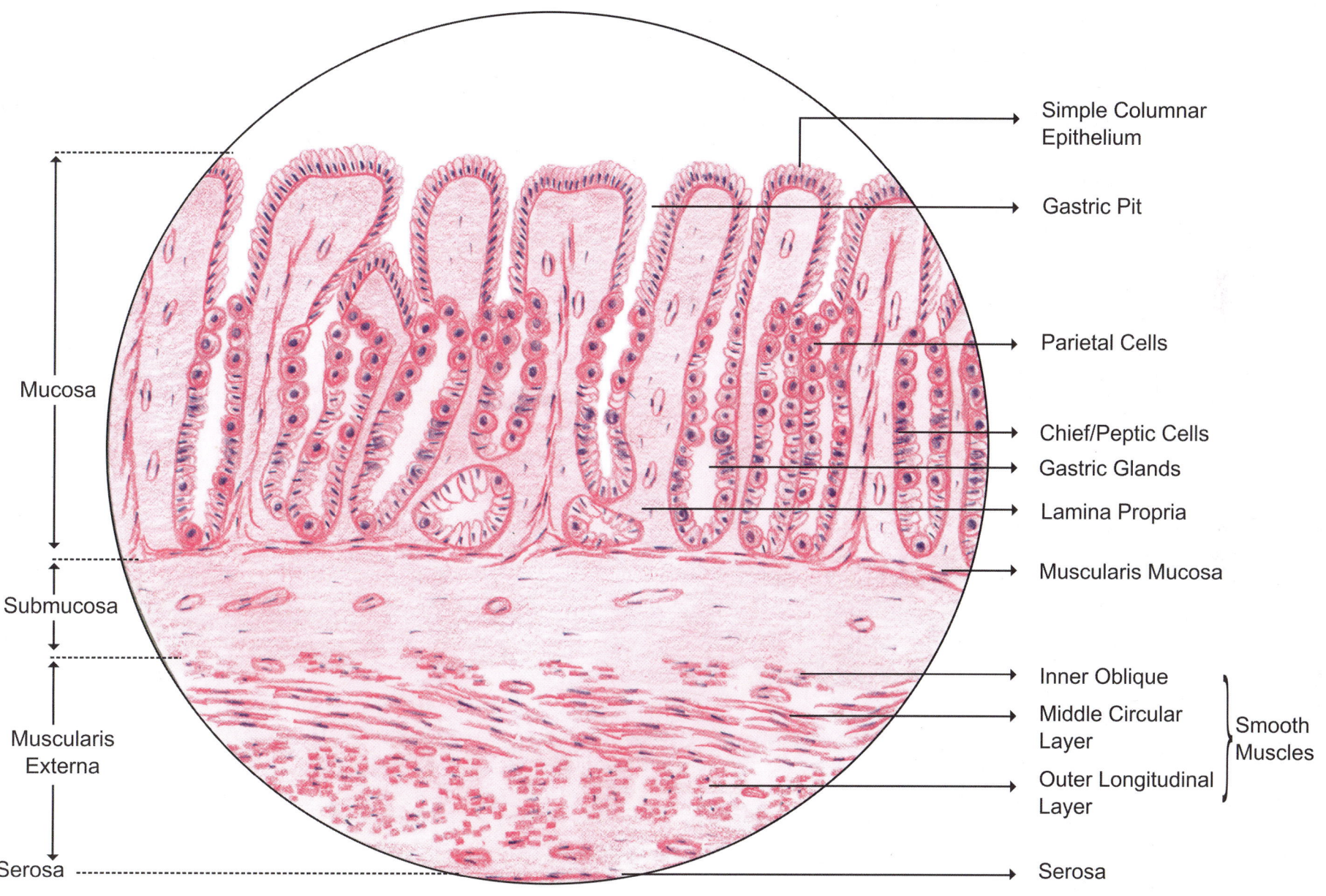

43. STOMACH: PYLORUS

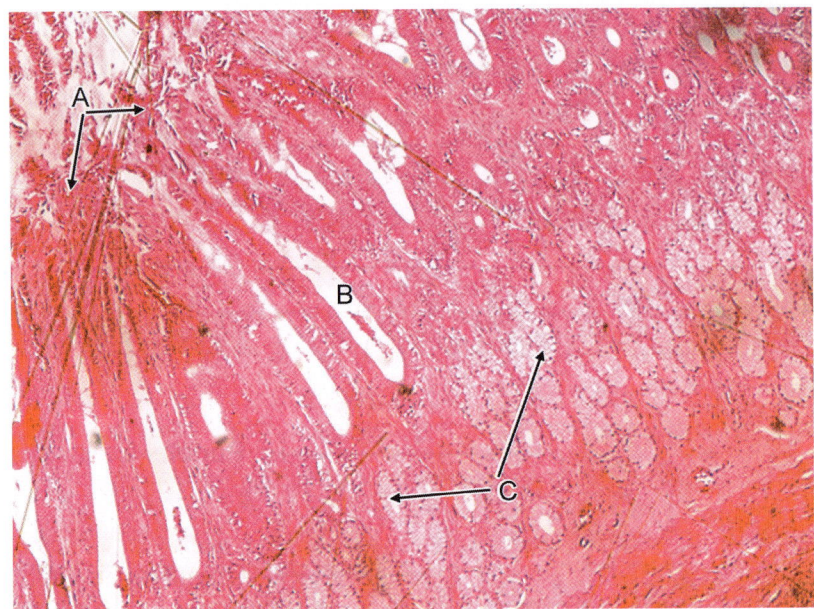

A	Simple Columnar Epithelium
B	Gastric Pits
C	Pyloric Glands

Identification Points

1. **Mucosal lining is simple columnar epithelium.**
2. **Deep gastric pits.**
3. **Lamina propria filled with coiled tubular glands.**

It has four layers—mucosa, submucosa, muscularis externa and serosa.

1. Mucosa:
   - Lining epithelium is simple columnar type. Shows depressions called gastric pits which are deeper occupying two-third of thickness of mucosa.
   - Lamina propria filled with pyloric glands which are coiled tubular type, open into base of pits.
   - Glands lined by mucous secreting cells, few parietal cells present.
   - Muscularis mucosae made of inner circular and outer longitudinal layers.
2. Submucosa—loose connective tissue with numerous blood vessels, lymphatics and nerve fibers.
3. Muscularis externa has three layers—inner oblique, middle circular, outer longitudinal smooth muscle.
4. Serosa—membrane made of a simple squamous epithelium.

43. STOMACH: PYLORUS

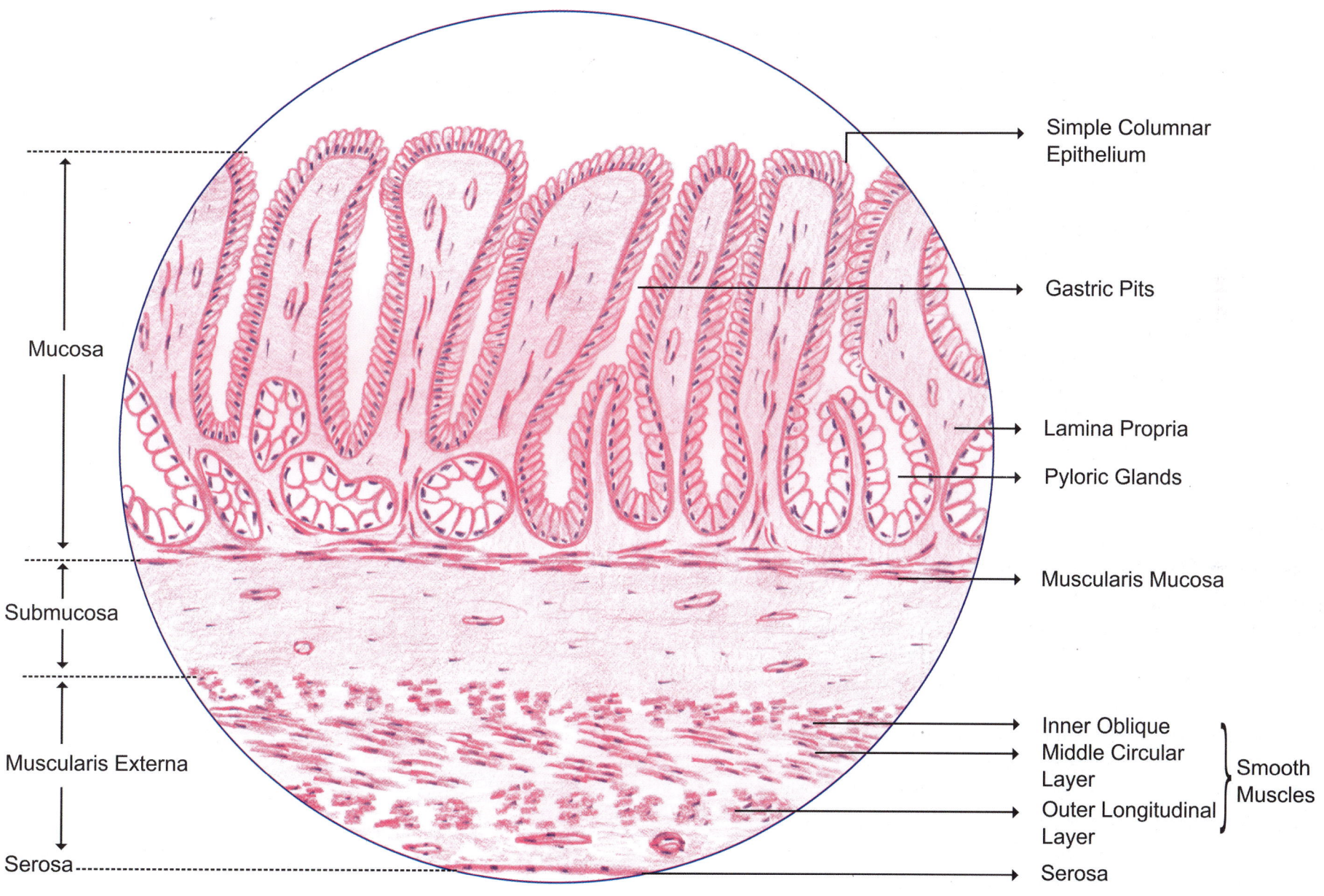

44. DUODENUM

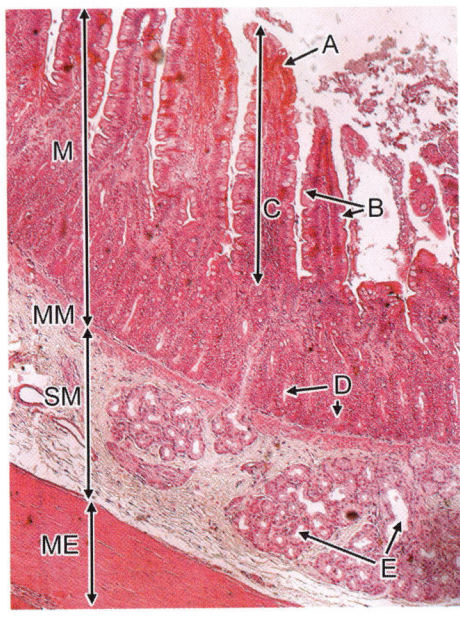

M	Mucosa
SM	Submucosa
ME	Muscularis Externa
MM	Muscularis Mucosa
A	Columnar Epithelium with Microvilli
C	Villus
D	Crypts of Lieberkühn
B	Goblet Cell
E	Brunner's Glands

Identification Points

1. **Mucosal villi, lined by columnar epithelium with microvilli (brush border) and goblet cells.**
2. **Submucosal Brunner's glands present.**

It has four layers—mucosa, submucosa, muscularis externa, adventitia/serosa.

1. Mucosa—lined by simple columnar cells with microvilli and goblet cells.
    - Mucosa thrown into folds called villi for increasing the surface area—broad tongue shaped.
    - Each villus has a core of lamina propria with a central lacteal and blood vessels.
    - Lamina propria filled with intestinal glands—crypts of Lieberkühn.
    - Cells present are columnar cells for absorption—enterocytes.
    - Mucus secreting goblet cells, paneth cells which secrete lysozymes, undifferentiated cells and neuroendocrine cells.
    - Muscularis mucosae made of inner circular and outer longitudinal smooth muscle layers.
2. Submucosa—loose connective tissue with numerous blood vessels, lymphatics and nerve fibers.
    Also contains tubuloalveolar mucus glands called as Brunner's glands. The secretions from the glands help in neutralizing the acidic contents from the stomach.
3. Muscularis externa—inner circular, outer longitudinal smooth muscle.
4. Serosa—peritoneal covering made of flat squamous cells. Areas not covered with the serous membrane contains only loose connective tissue called adventitia.

44. DUODENUM

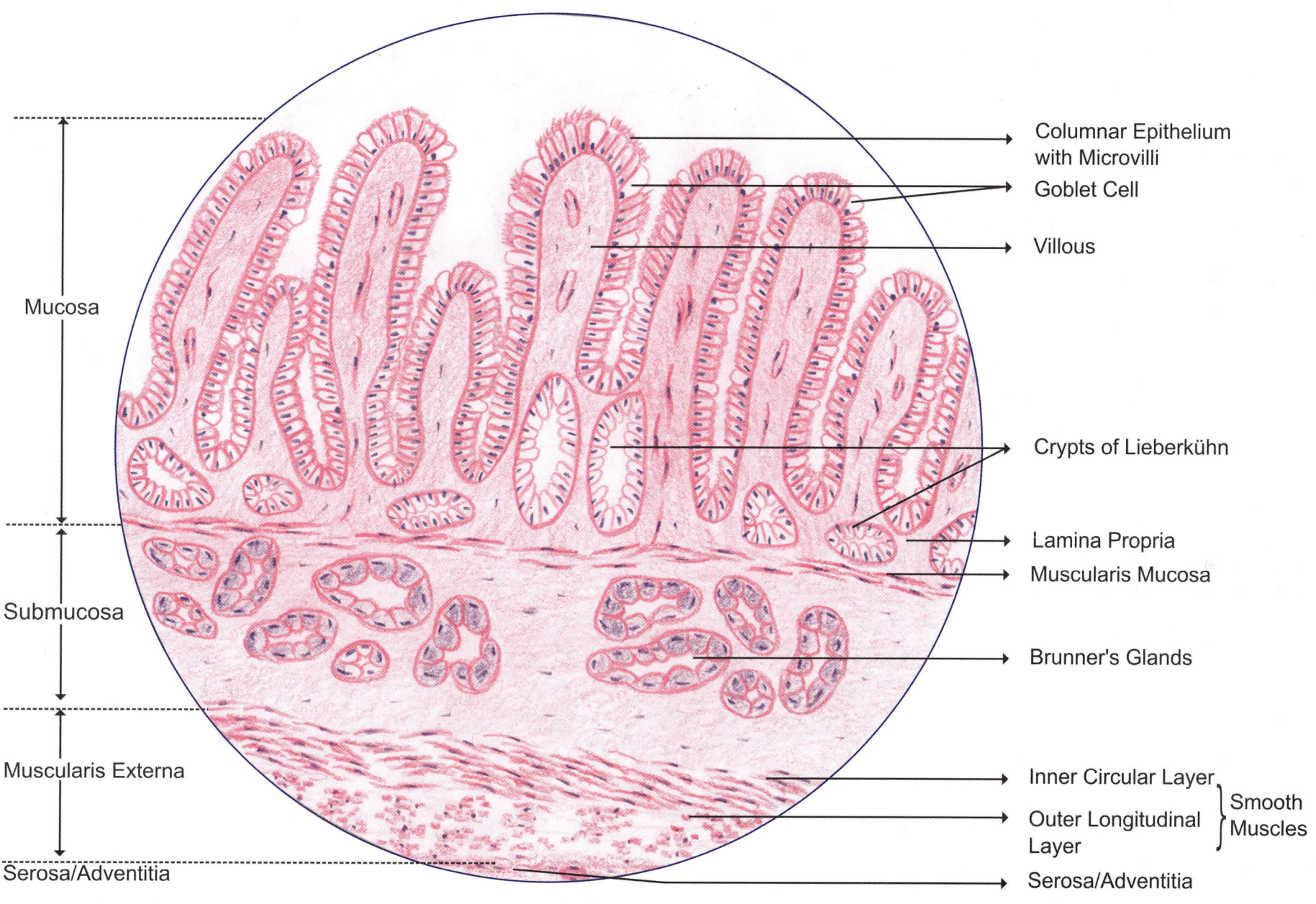

45. JEJUNUM

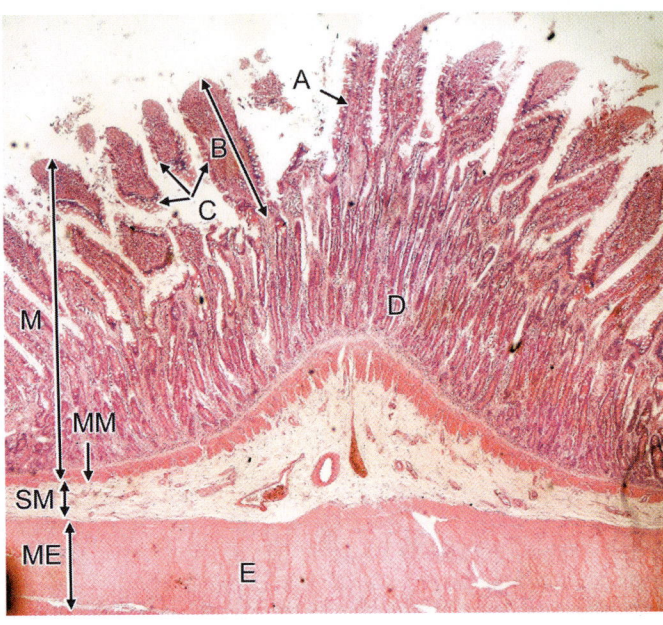

M	Mucosa
SM	Submucosa
ME	Muscularis Externa
MM	Muscularis Mucosa
A	Columnar Epithelium with Microvilli
B	Villus
D	Crypts of Lieberkühn
C	Goblet Cell
E	Smooth Muscles

Identification Points

1. **Mucosal villi, lined by columnar epithelium with microvilli (brush border) and lots of goblet cells.**
2. **Intestinal glands (crypts of Lieberkühn) present.**
3. **No submucosal glands or Peyer's patch.**

It has four layers—mucosa, submucosa, muscularis externa, serosa.
1. Mucosa—lined by simple columnar cells with microvilli and goblet cells.
   – Mucosa thrown into folds called villi for increasing the surface area—tall leaf shaped.
   – Each villus has a core of lamina propria with a central lacteal and blood vessels.
   – Lamina propria filled with intestinal glands—crypts of Lieberkühn.
   – Cells present are columnar cells for absorption—enterocytes.
   – Mucus secreting goblet cells, paneth cells which secrete lysozymes, undifferentiated cells and neuroendocrine cells.
   – Muscularis mucosae made of inner circular and outer longitudinal layers of smooth muscles.
2. Submucosa—loose connective tissue with numerous blood vessels, lymphatics and nerve fibers.
3. Muscularis externa—inner circular, outer longitudinal smooth muscle.
4. Serosa—peritoneal covering made of flat squamous cells.

45. JEJUNUM

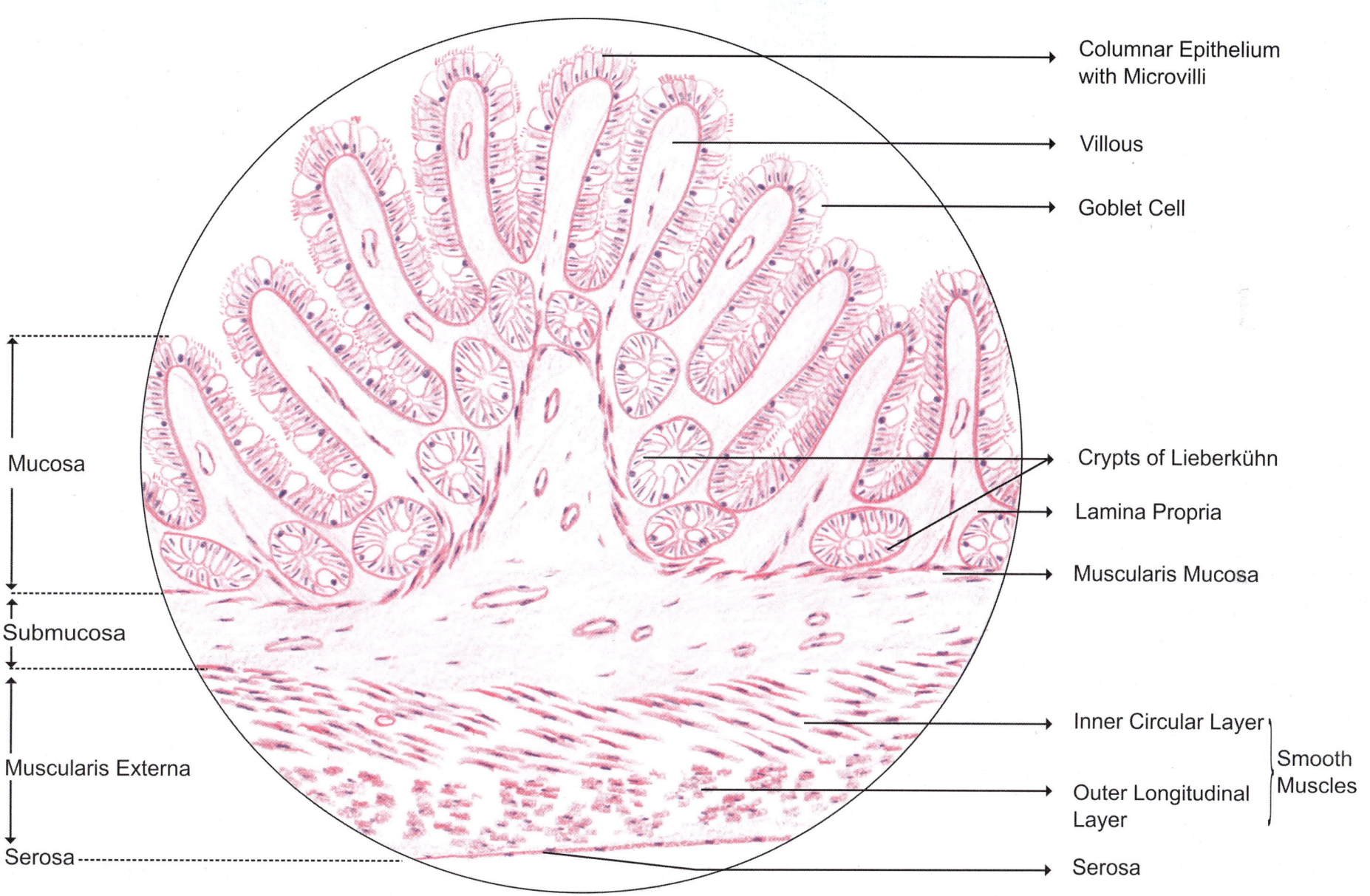

46. ILEUM

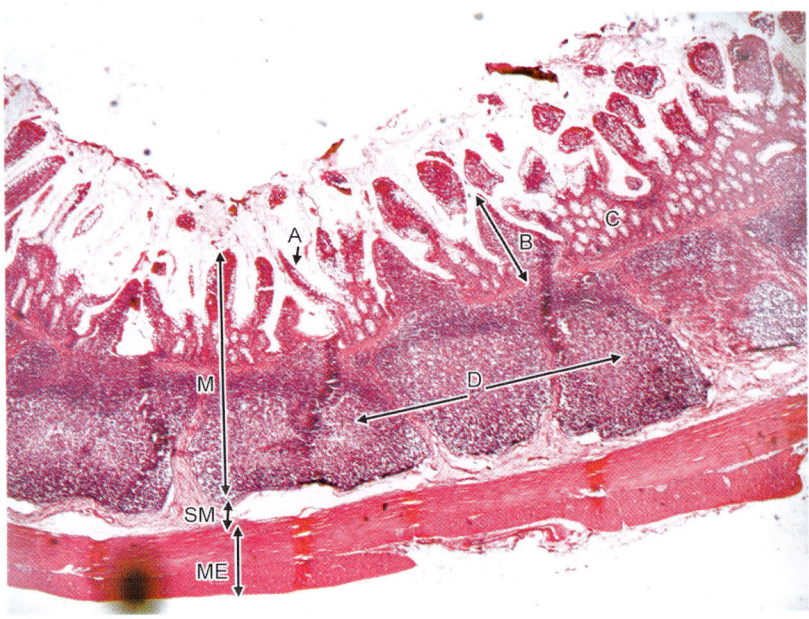

M	Mucosa
SM	Submucosa
ME	Muscularis Externa
A	Columnar Epithelium with Microvilli
B	Villus
C	Crypts of Lieberkühn
D	Peyer's Patch

Identification Points

1. **Mucosal villi, lined by columnar epithelium with microvilli (brush border) and lots of goblet cells.**
2. **Peyer's patch in mucosal layer extending to submucosa.**

It has four layers—mucosa, submucosa, muscularis externa, serosa.

1. Mucosa—lined by simple columnar cells with microvilli and goblet cells.
   Mucosa thrown into folds called villi for increasing the surface area—small finger like.
   – Each villus has a core of lamina propria with a central lacteal and blood vessels.
   – Lamina propria filled with intestinal glands—crypts of Lieberkühn.
   – Cells present are columnar cells for absorption—enterocytes.
   – Mucus secreting goblet cells, paneth cells which secrete lysozymes, undifferentiated cells and neuroendocrine cells.
   – Lamina propria shows aggregations of lymphoid follicles called Peyer's patches each containing 10–200 follicles.
   – Muscularis mucosae made of inner circular and outer longitudinal layers of smooth muscles.
2. Submucosa—loose connective tissue with numerous blood vessels, lymphatics and nerve fibers.
3. Muscularis externa—inner circular, outer longitudinal smooth muscle.
4. Serosa—peritoneal covering made of flat squamous cells.

46. ILEUM

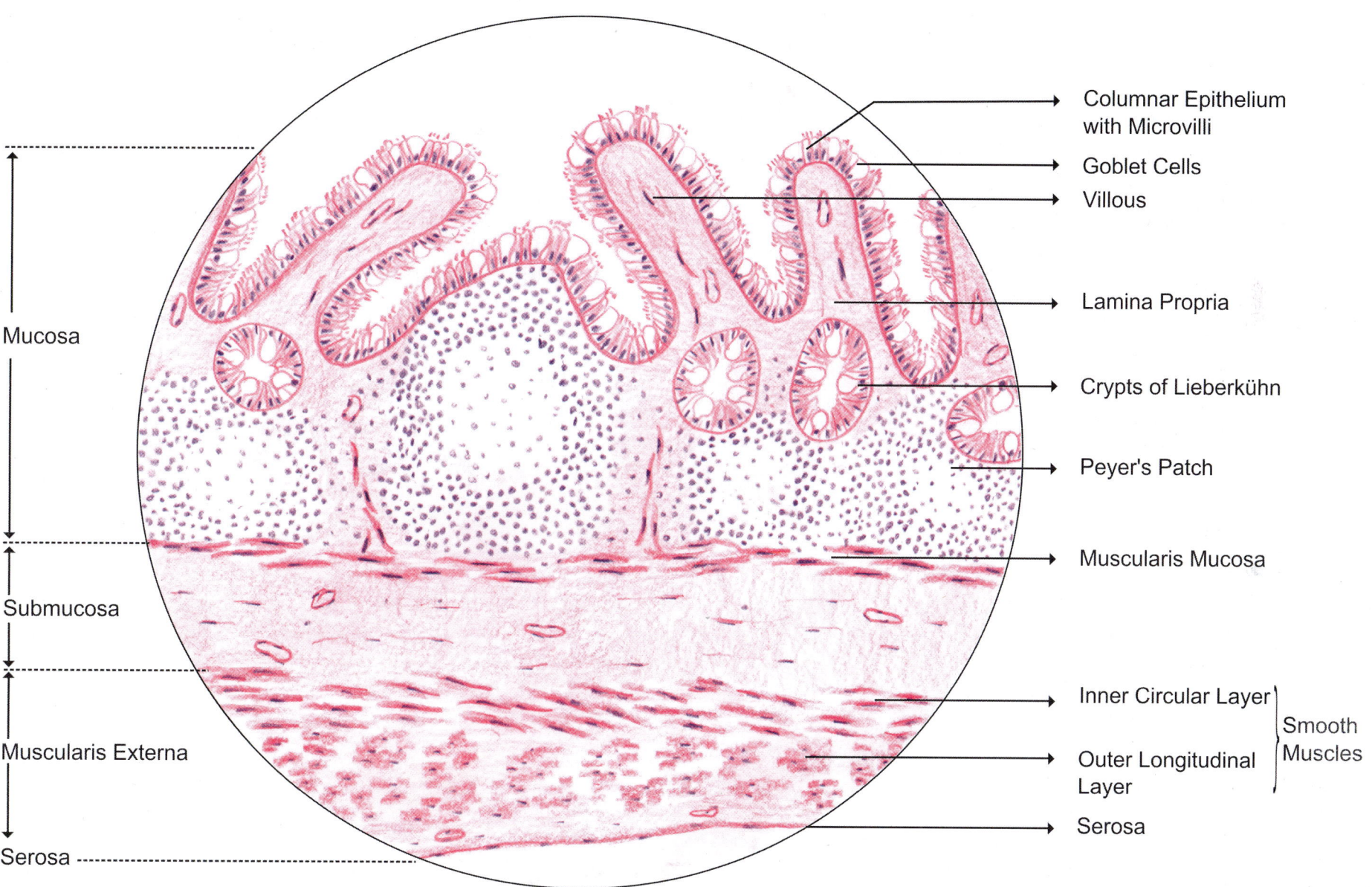

47. LARGE INTESTINE

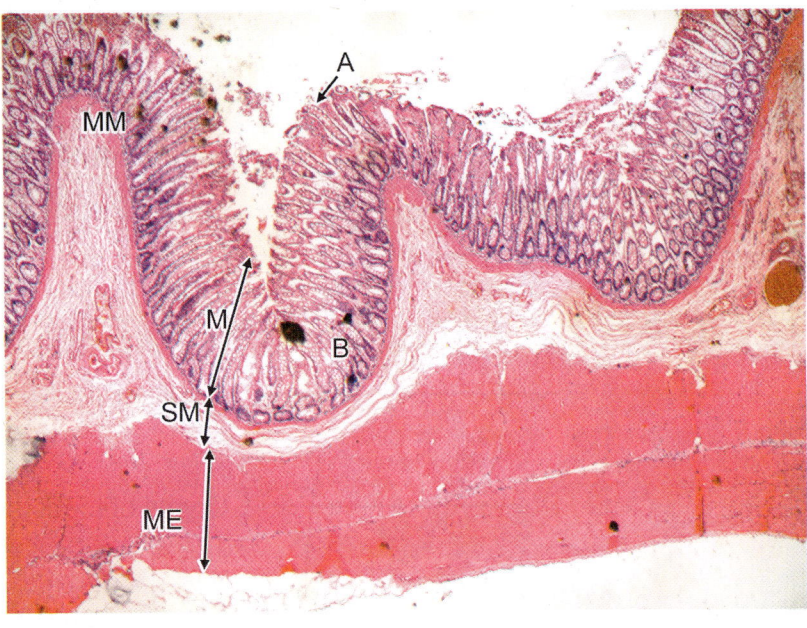

M	Mucosa
SM	Submucosa
ME	Muscularis Externa
MM	Muscularis Mucosa
A	Columnar Epithelium with Microvilli
B	Crypts of Lieberkühn

Identification Points

1. Lining epithelium is tall columnar with lots of goblet cells.
2. Lamina propria filled with crypts of Lieberkühn.
3. Taenia coli in the muscularis externa.

It has four layers—mucosa, submucosa, muscularis externa, adventitia/serosa
1. Mucosa—lined by simple columnar cells with microvilli. Goblet cells are numerous.
   – No villi are seen.
   – Lamina propria filled with intestinal glands—crypts of Lieberkühn.
   – Cells present are columnar cells for absorption, mucus secreting goblet cells, undifferentiated cells and neuroendocrine cells. No paneth cells.
   – Solitary lymphoid follicles are seen.
   – Muscularis mucosae made of inner circular and outer longitudinal layers of smooth muscles.
2. Submucosa—loose connective tissue with numerous blood vessels, lymphatics and nerve fibers.
3. Muscularis externa—inner circular, outer longitudinal smooth muscle.
   – Outer longitudinal layer is thickened at three areas forming taenia coli.
4. Serosa—peritoneal covering made of flat squamous cells. Adventitia—connective tissue in areas not covered by peritoneum.

47. LARGE INTESTINE

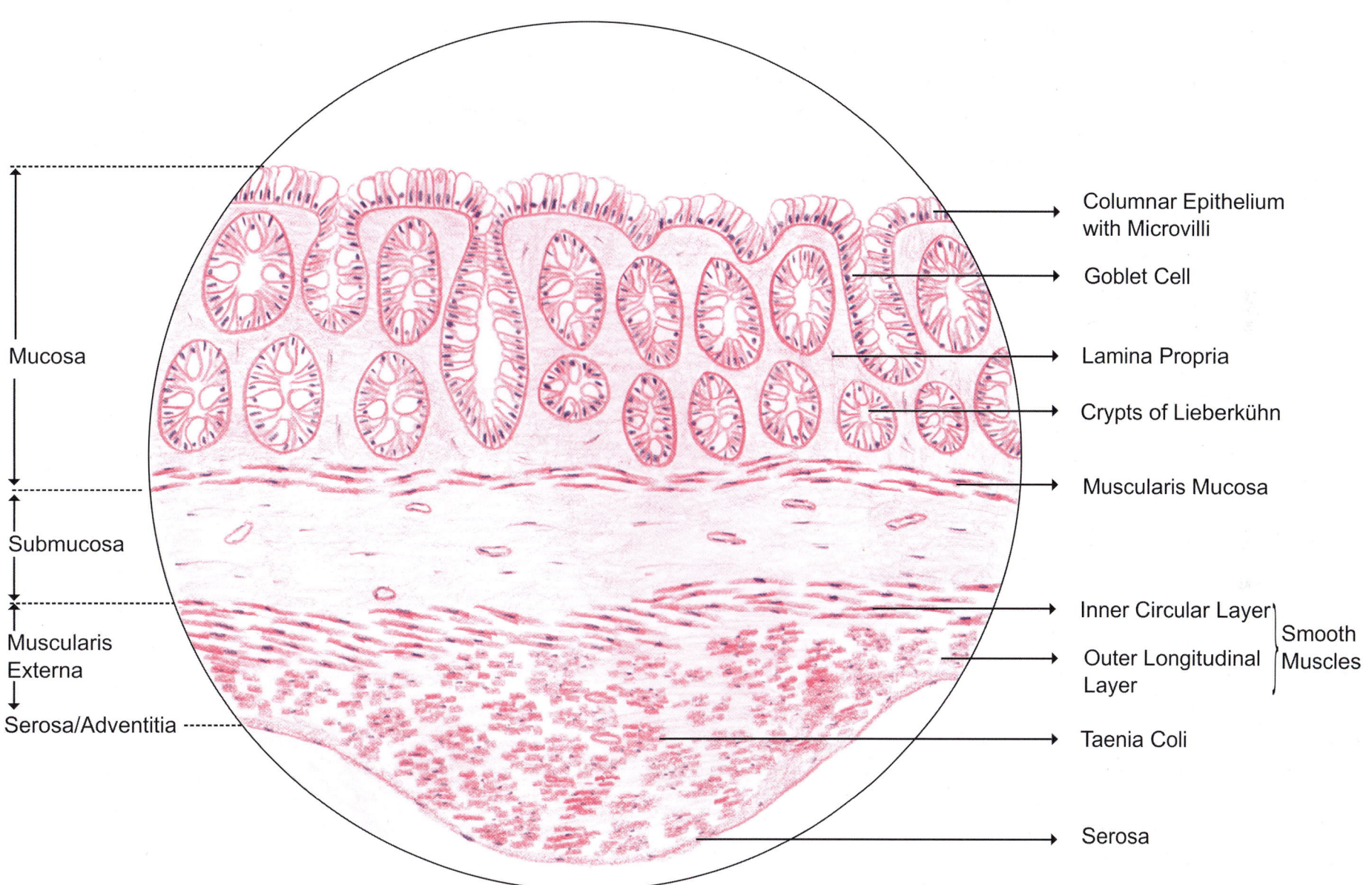

48. APPENDIX

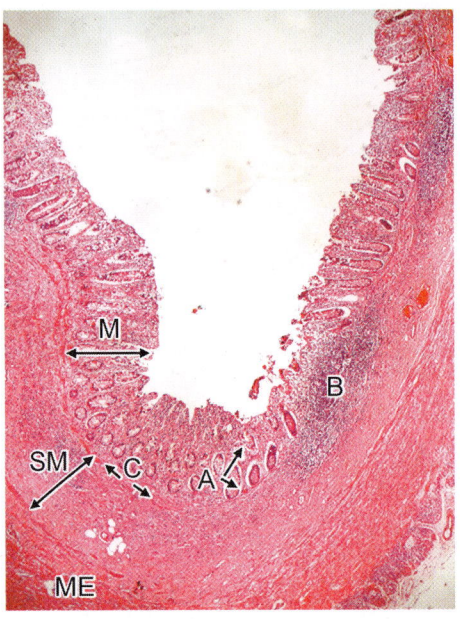

M	Mucosa
SM	Submucosa
ME	Muscularis Externa
C	Muscularis Mucosa (Discontinuous)
A	Crypts of Lieberkühn
B	Lymphoid Follicle

Identification Points

1. **Lining epithelium is tall columnar with lots of goblet cells.**
2. **Lamina propria filled with lymphoid follicles and few crypts of Lieberkühn.**
3. **No villi, no taenia coli.**

It has four layers—mucosa, submucosa, muscularis externa, serosa.
1. Mucosa—lined by simple columnar cells with microvilli. Goblet cells are numerous.
   – Lamina propria contains few intestinal glands—crypts of Lieberkühn.
   – It also contains numerous lymphoid follicles which extend into submucosa and bulge into the lumen making it irregularly narrow.
   – Muscularis mucosa is discontinuous.
2. Submucosa—loose connective tissue with numerous blood vessels, lymphatics and nerve fibers. Also contains lymphoid aggregates which has extended from mucosa.
3. Muscularis externa—inner circular, outer longitudinal smooth muscle.
4. Serosa—peritoneal covering made of flat squamous cells.

48. APPENDIX

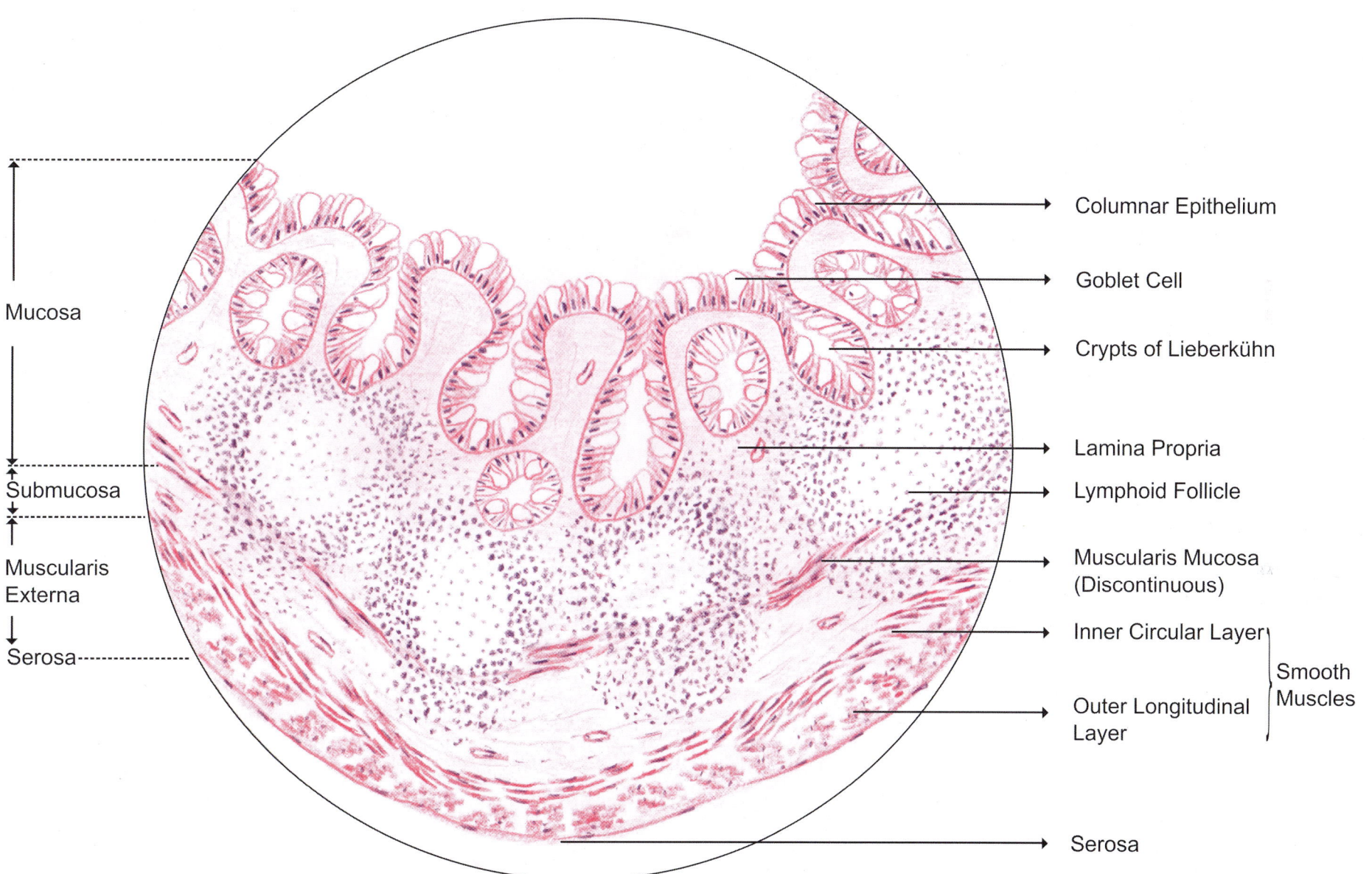

49. LIVER

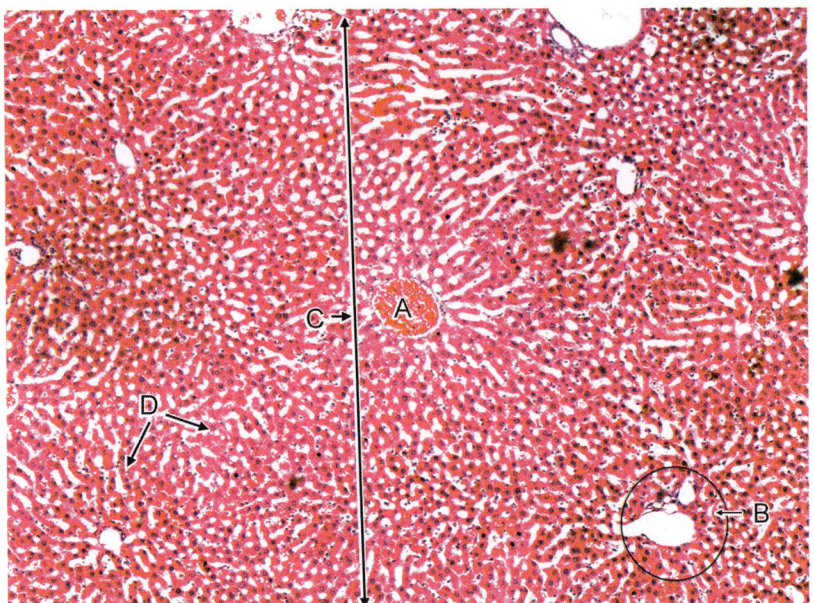

C	Hexagonal Hepatic Lobule
B	Portal Triad
D	Hepatocytes in Radiating Cords
A	Central Vein

Identification Points

1. Hexagonal-shaped hepatic lobules with central vein and radiating hepatocytes with sinusoids in between seen.
2. Portal triad—containing branch of portal vein, hepatic artery and bile ductule present at the corners of lobules seen.

- Connective tissue capsule sends septa inside and divide the parenchyma into lobules.
- Classical liver lobule is hexagonal in shape.
- At the center it contains a central vein with branching and anastomosing plates of hepatocytes radiating outwards. These plates of hepatocytes are separated by sinusoids.
- At the periphery of the lobule portal triads are present which contain branches of hepatic artery and portal vein with bile ductules.
- Hepatocytes are polyhedral in shape with round nuclei. Sinusoids lined by endothelial cells. Also contains phagocytic macrophages called Kupffer cells.
- The flow of blood is from portal triad towards the central vein whereas the flow of bile is towards the periphery of the lobules.
- Portal lobule—hexagonal lobule with portal triad at the center and central veins at the periphery.
- Portal acinus—the area between two adjacent central veins with the central axis formed by the branch of hepatic artery and portal vein.

49. LIVER

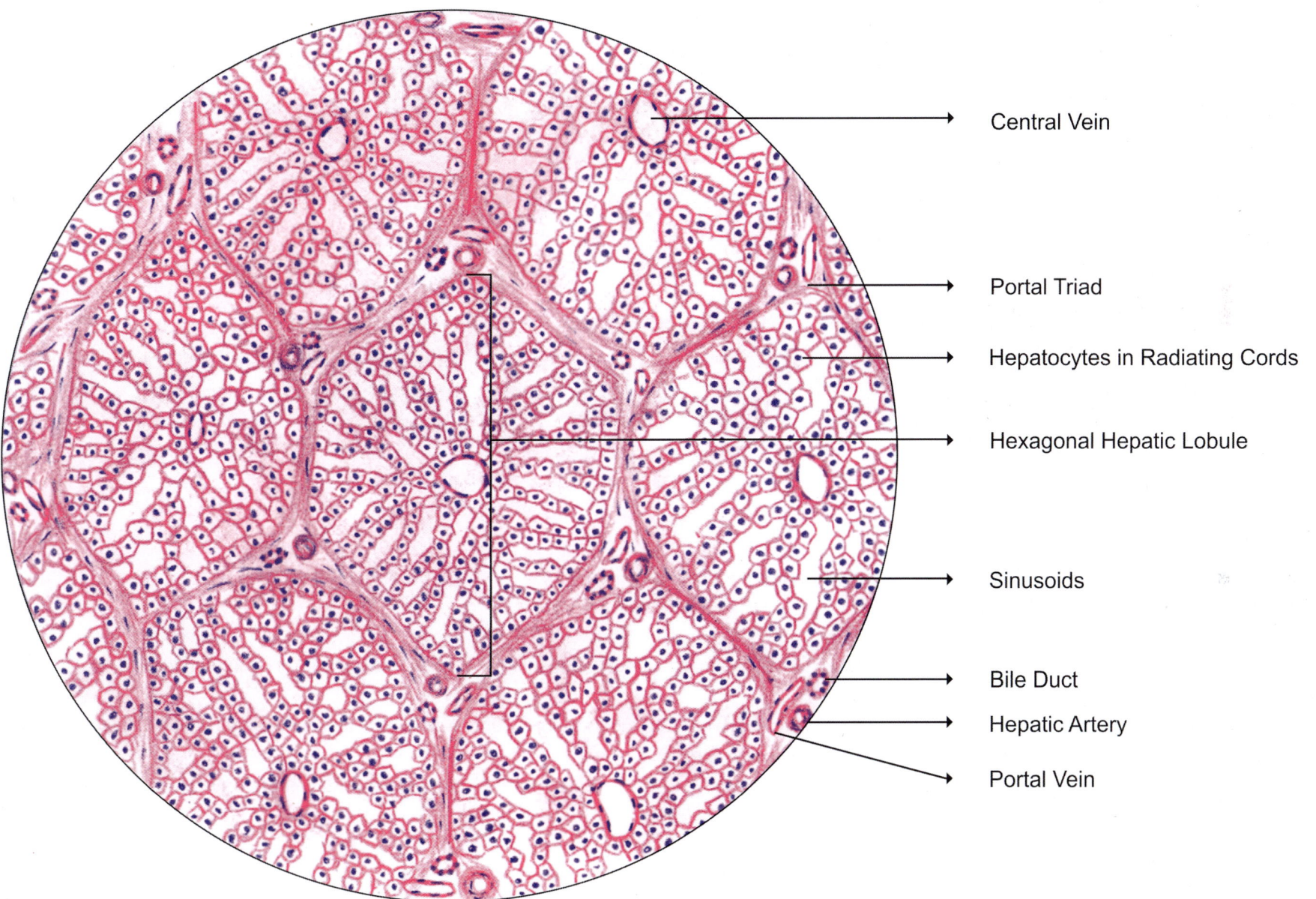

50. GALLBLADDER

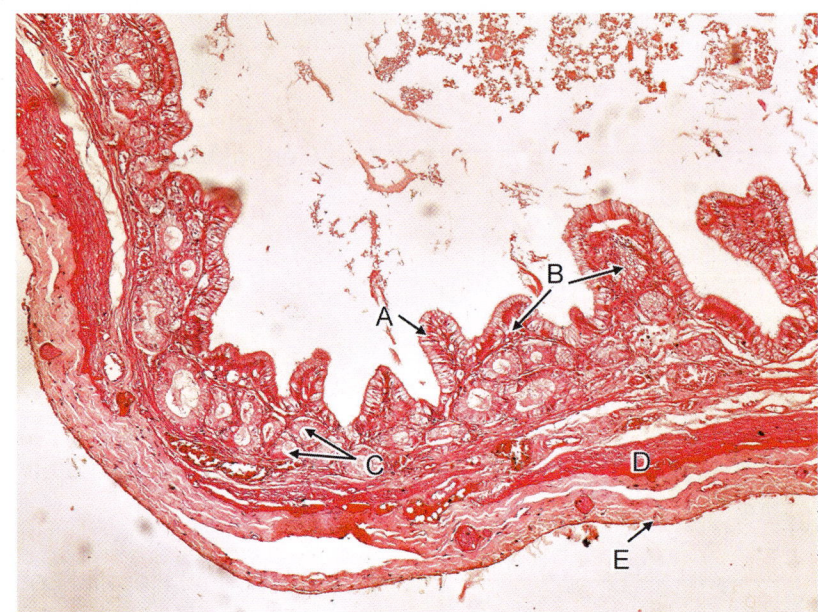

D	Fibromuscular Layer
E	Serosa/Adventitia
A	Columnar Epithelium with Microvilli
B	Mucosal Folds
C	Crypt

Identification Points

1. **Mucosa thrown into folds lined by simple tall columnar epithelium with brush border.**
2. **Fibromuscular wall seen.**

- There are extensive mucosal fold into the lumen which allows the distension of bladder and increase the surface area for absorption (concentration of bile).
- Gallbladder is a three layered structure.
    1. Mucosal layer—lined by simple tall columnar epithelium lying over a layer of lamina propria. Columnar cells have apical microvilli which help in absorption.
    2. Fibromuscular layer—made of connective tissue and smooth muscles fibers.
    3. Outer layer of serosa—peritoneal covering made of flat squamous cells. Areas not covered with the serous membrane contain only loose connective tissue called adventitia.

50. GALLBLADDER

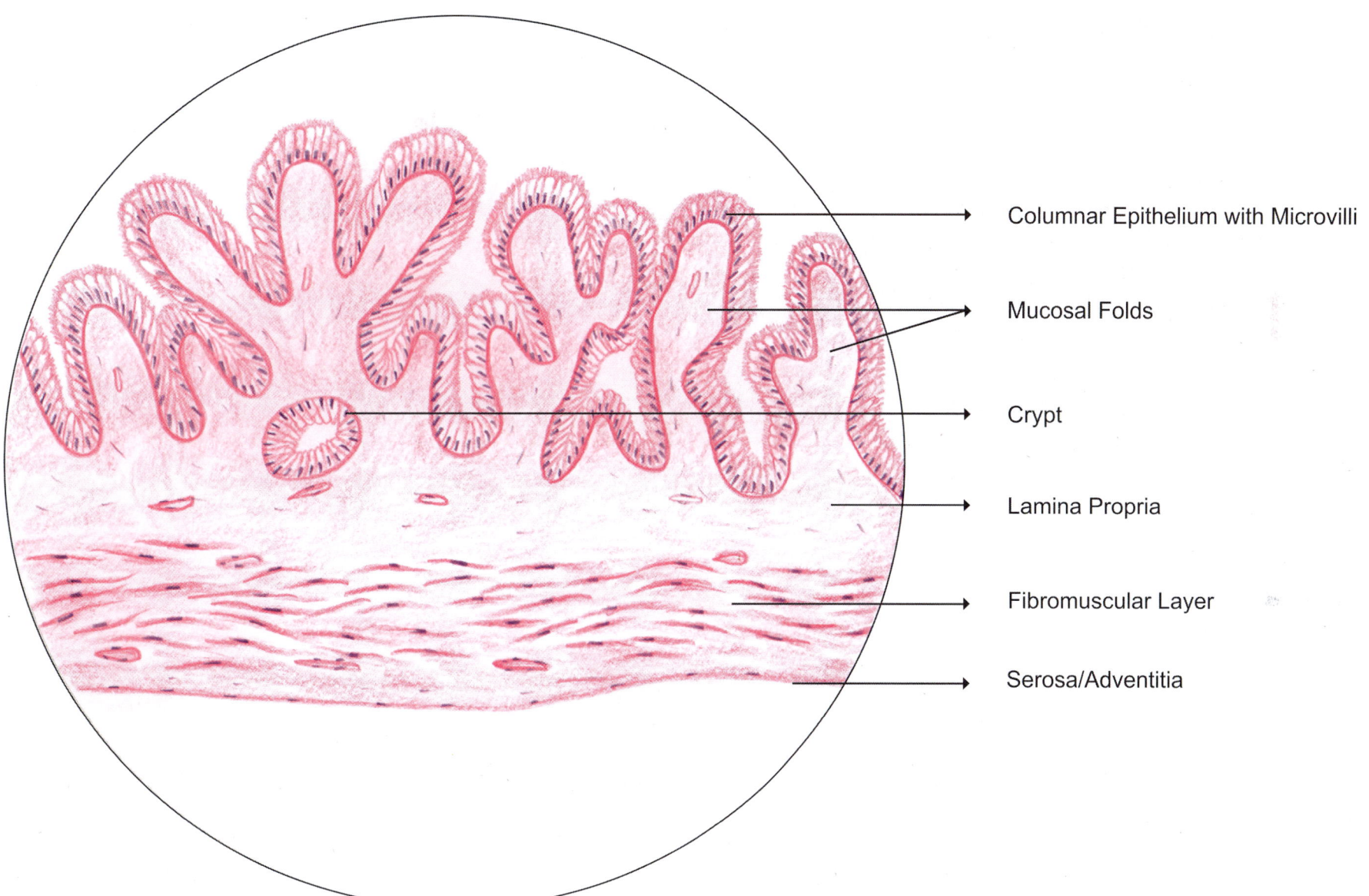

51. PANCREAS

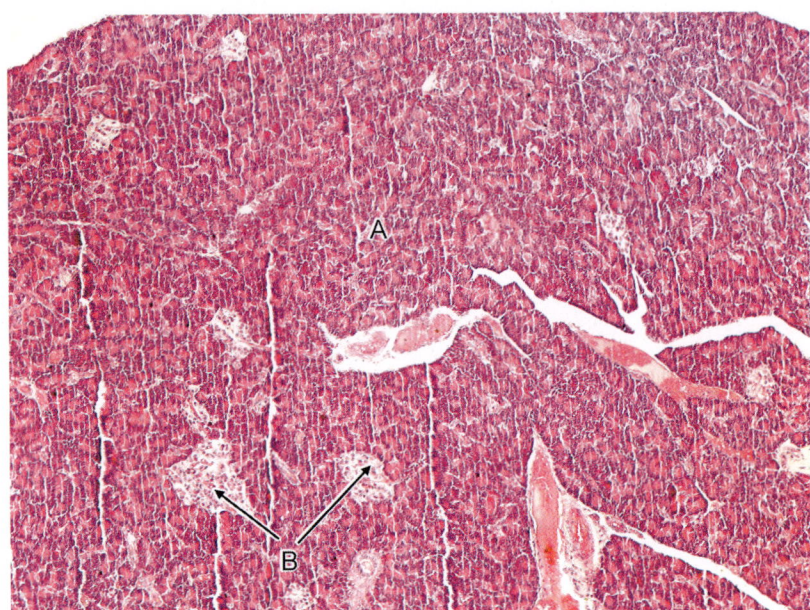

A	Serous Acini
B	Islets of Langerhans

Identification Points

1. **Serous acini with biphasic stain and centroacinar cells.**
2. **Islets of Langerhans seen.**

- Pancreas is an exo-endocrine gland.
- It has thin capsule, septa from capsule divides gland into lobules.
- Pancreatic acini are compactly arranged.
- Biphasic stain more pronounced, apical portion of cell cytoplasm is eosinophilic (zymogen granules) and basal portion is basophilic.
- Centroacinar cells are the beginning of the intercalated ducts which are seen at the center of the acini.
- Islets of Langerhans forms endocrine part of gland. Highly vascular.
  - It consists of polyhedral cells which are of three types—alpha, beta, delta.
  - Beta cells form 70% of islets, located in the center and secrete insulin.
  - Alpha cells make 20%, located peripherally and secrete glucagon.
  - Delta cells secrete stomatostatin.

51. PANCREAS

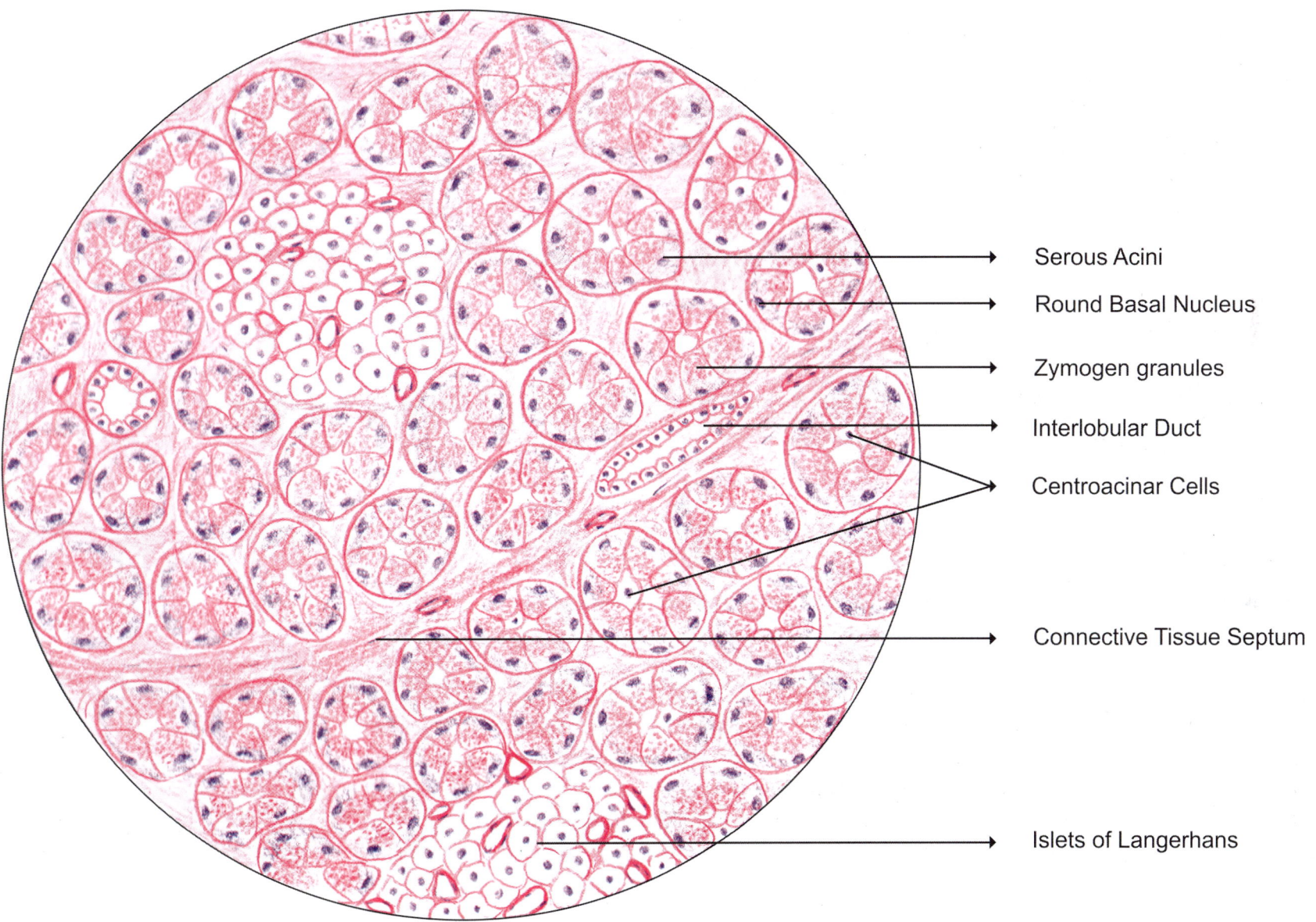

52. KIDNEY

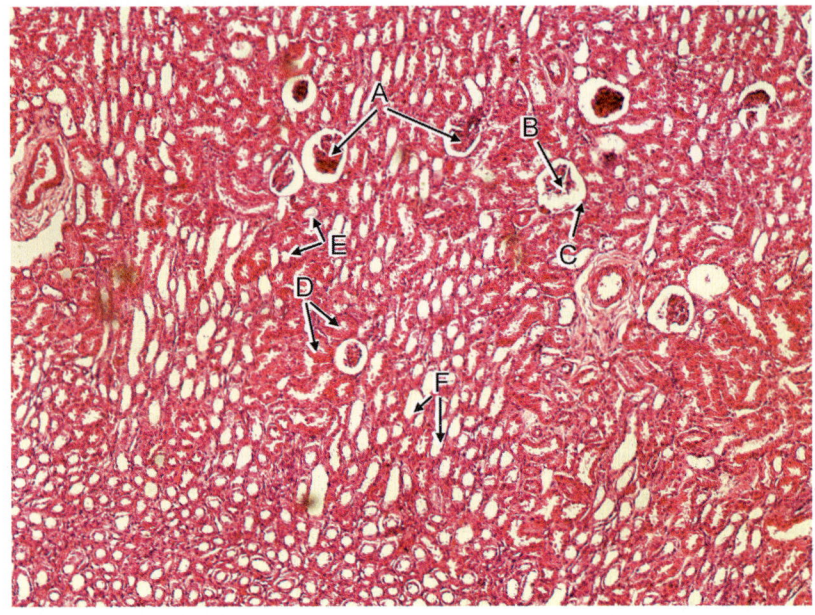

A	Renal Corpuscle
B	Glomerulus
C	Bowman's Capsule
D	Proximal Convoluted Tubule
E	Distal Convoluted Tubule
F	Collecting Duct

Identification Points

1. **Outer cortex—renal corpuscles and sections of proximal and distal convoluted tubules seen.**
2. **Inner medulla—sections of collecting ducts and loop of Henle seen.**

- Outer cortex, inner medulla seen.
- Cortex contains renal corpuscles—Bowman's capsule with glomerular plexus. Their function is filtration from plasma.
- Section of proximal convoluted tubules—eosinophilic columnar cells with brush border, narrow lumen.
- Section of distal convoluted tubules—pale staining cuboidal cells, large lumen
- Medulla contains sections of collecting ducts and loops of Henle lined by cuboidal cells and squamous cells.
- Functional unit of kidney is the nephron. It consists of renal corpuscles, proximal convoluted tubules, distal convoluted tubules and loop of Henle.

52. KIDNEY

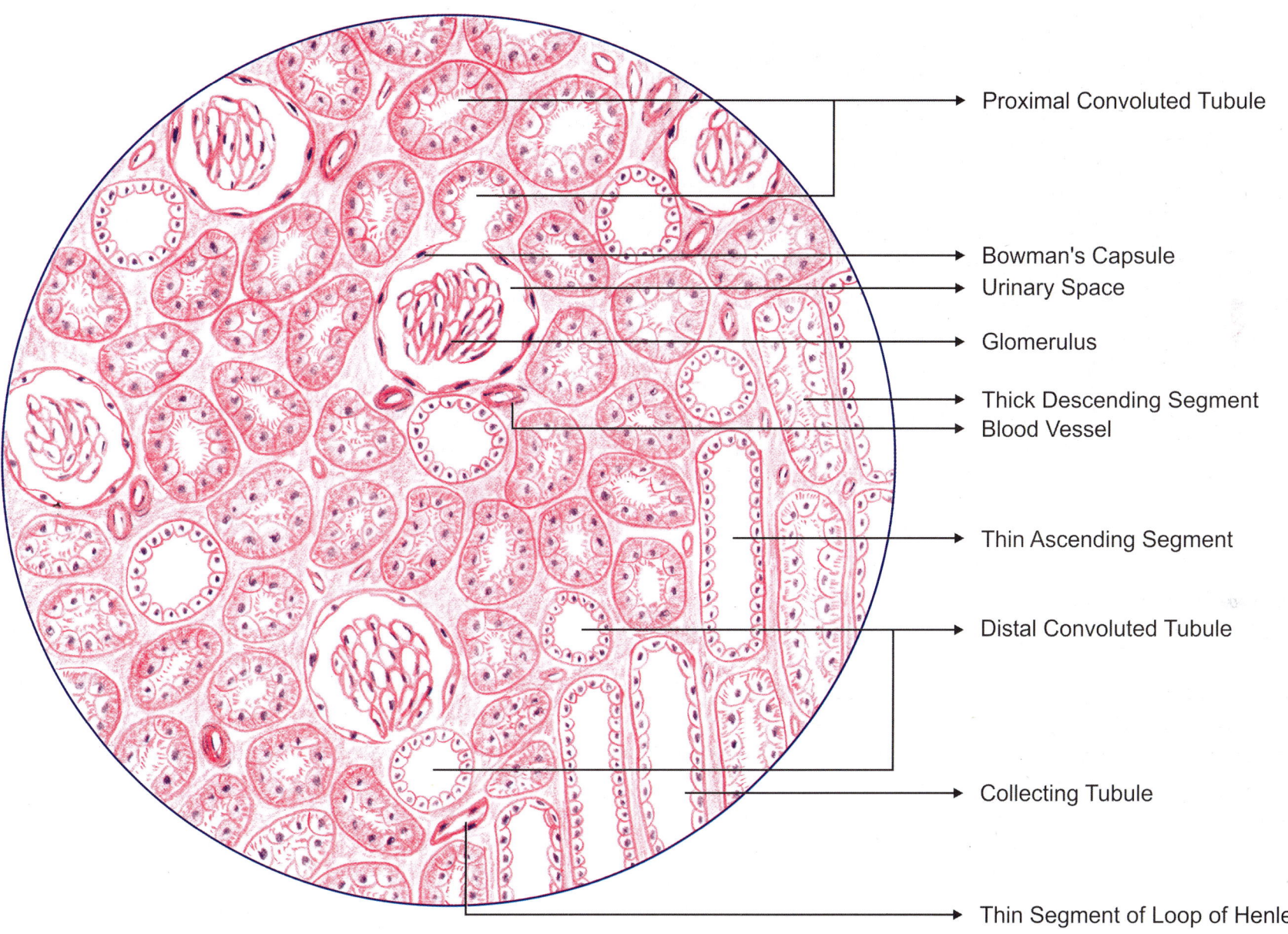

53. URETER

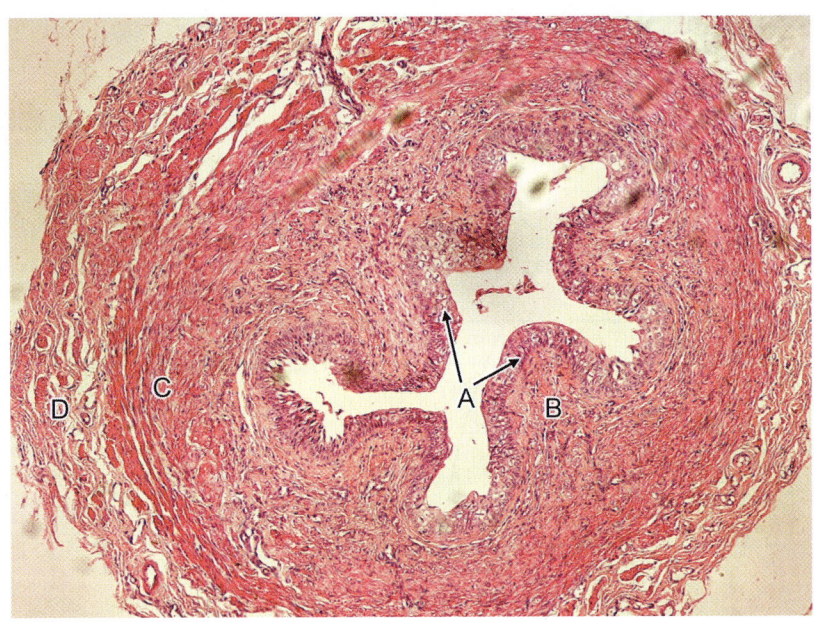

A	Transitional Epithelium
B	Lamina Propria
C	Layer of Smooth Muscles
D	Adventitia/Serosa

Identification Points

1. **Mucosal folds lined by transitional epithelium.**
2. **Muscular tube—inner longitudinal, outer circular layer of smooth muscles.**

1. Mucosa shows longitudinal folds—lumen is star shaped, lined by transitional epithelium.
   – Epithelium rests on layer of lamina propria.
2. Thick middle muscle layer—inner longitudinal, outer circular layer of smooth muscles.
3. Outer layer of loose connective tissue with blood vessels.

53. URETER

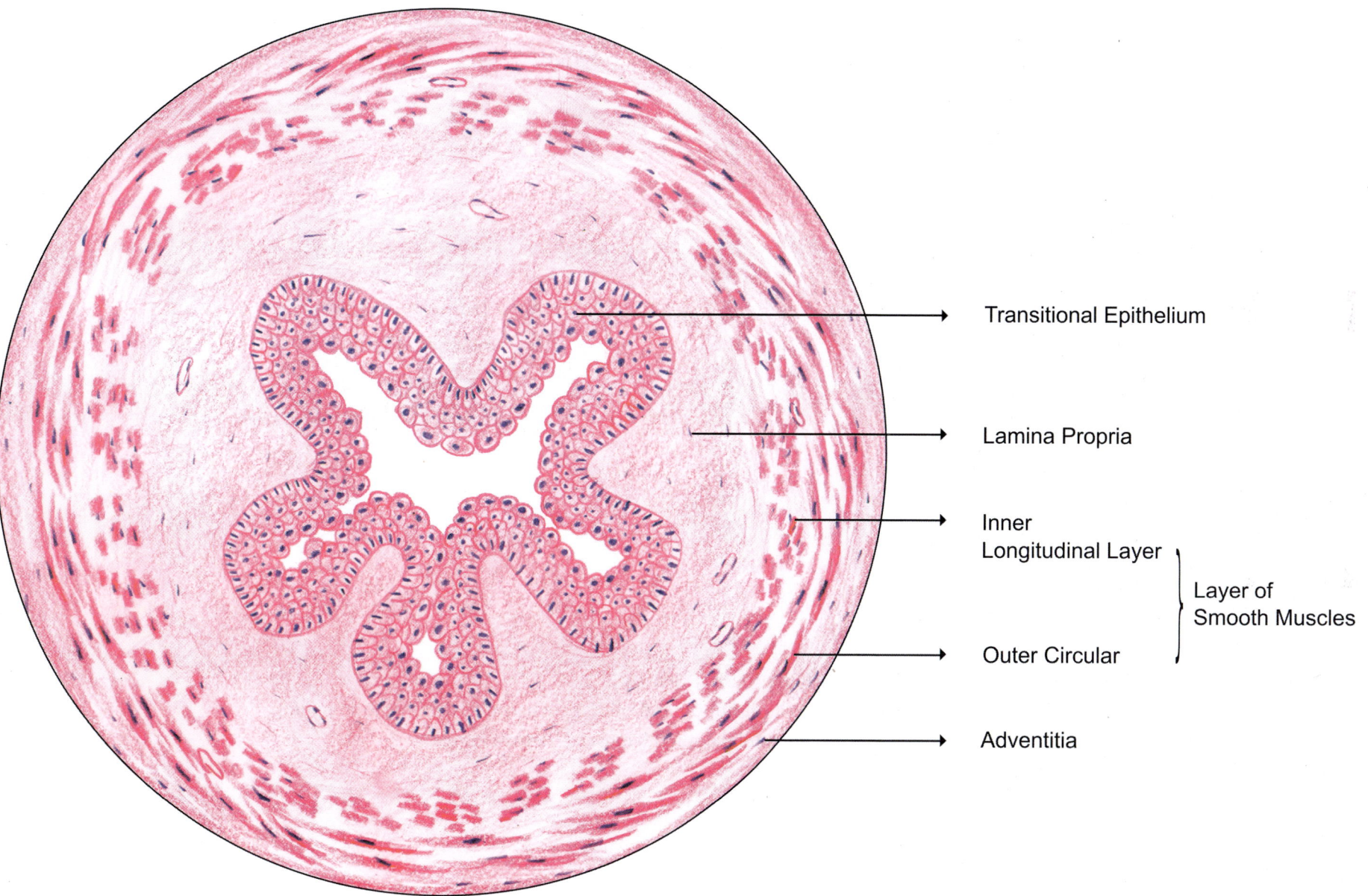

54. URINARY BLADDER

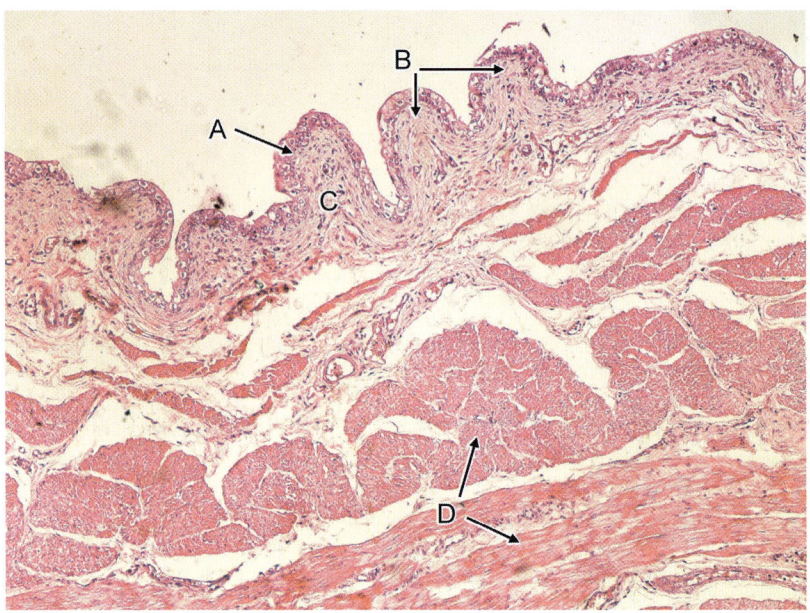

A	Transitional Epithelium
B	Mucosal Folds
C	Lamina Propria
D	Layer of Smooth Muscles

Identification Points

1. **Mucosa lined by transitional epithelium.**
2. **Thick muscular wall made of three ill-defined layers.**
3. **Thick lamina propria.**

1. Mucosa lined by transitional epithelium resting over thick layer of loose connective tissue.
    – Empty bladder mucosa is thrown into folds. Distended bladder folds disappear and epithelium becomes thin due to stretching.
2. Thick muscle layer—inner longitudinal, middle circular and outer longitudinal smooth muscle—detrusor muscle.
3. Outer serosa—lined by flat squamous cells.

54. URINARY BLADDER

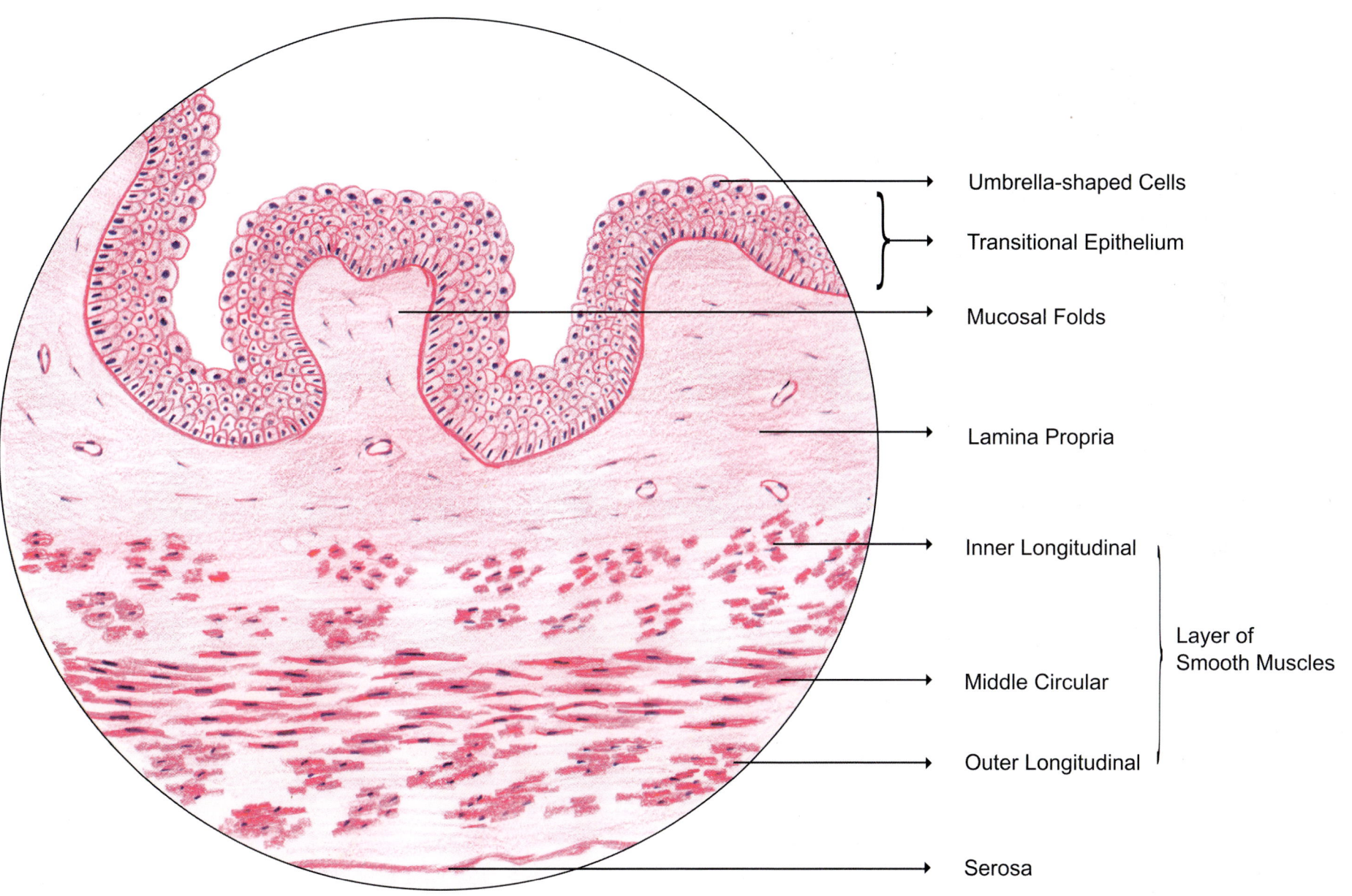

55. PROSTATIC URETHRA

Prostatic Urethra

- Section shows prostatic urethra surrounded by prostatic glands.
- Lumen of urethra is crescent shaped, lined by transitional epithelium.
- Posterior wall of urethra shows dome-shaped colliculus seminalis/verumontanum.
- Central part shows prostatic utricle lined by simple or psuedostratified columnar cells.
- Two ejaculatory ducts seen on either side of utricle.
- On each side of colliculus is the prostatic sinuses which contains the opening of the ducts of prostatic glands.
- Surrounding the urethra acini of prostatic glands and fibromuscular stroma is seen.

55. PROSTATIC URETHRA

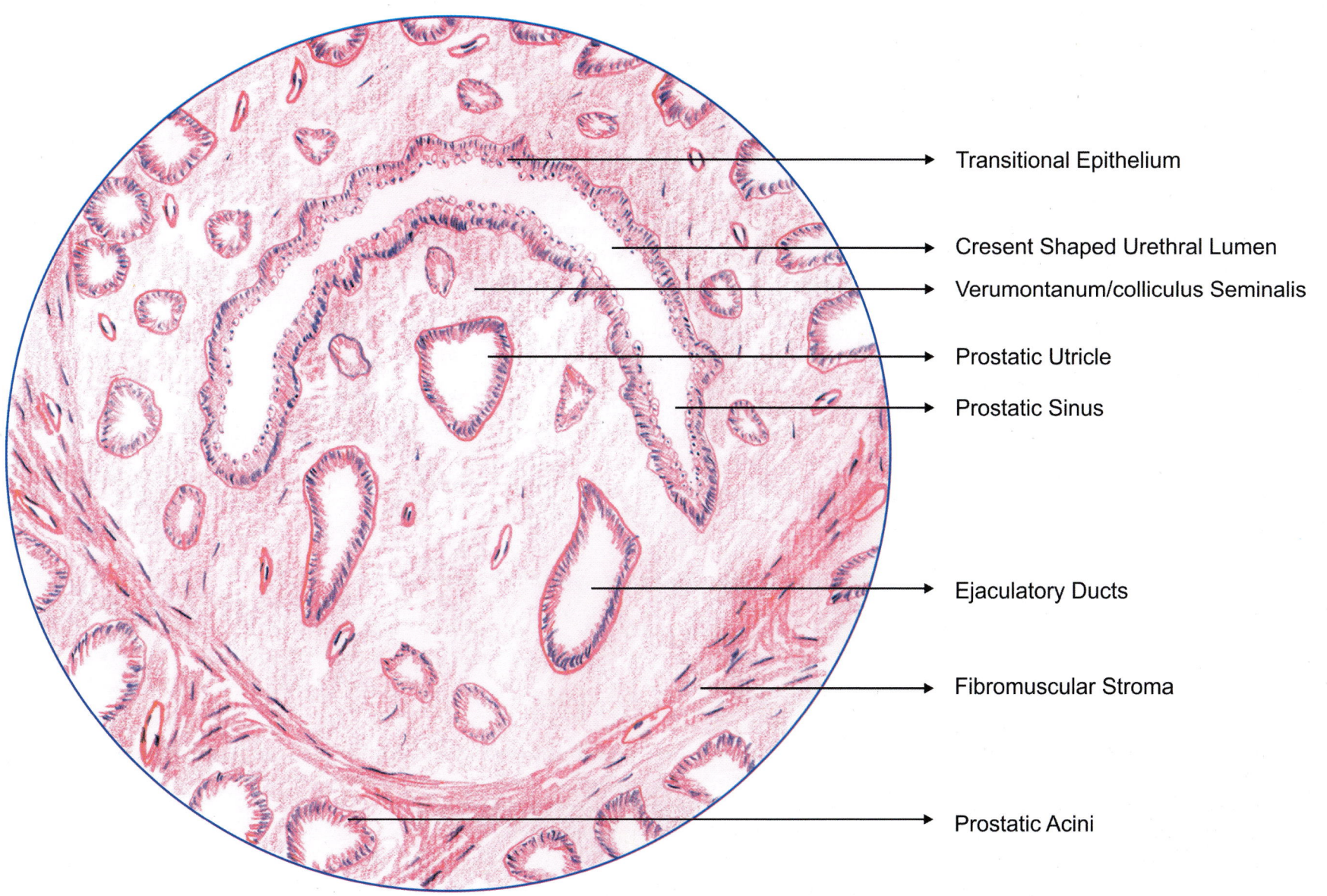

56. TESTIS

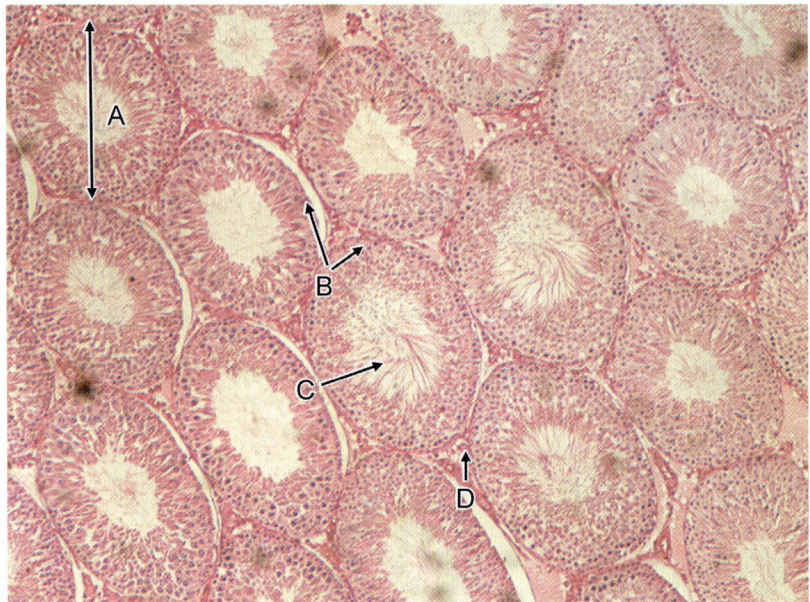

A	Seminiferous Tubule
B	Spermatogonia
C	Spermatozoa
D	Interstitial Cells of Leydig

Identification Points

1. Sections of seminiferous tubules lined by spermatogonia, different stages of spermatocytes and Sertoli cells.
2. Interstitial cells of Leydig in between the tubules seen.

- Connective tissue covering—tunica albuginea.
- Sections of seminiferous tubules with many layers of cells seen.
- Lined by cells of different stages of spermatogenesis and Sertoli cells.
- Sertoli cells/sustentacular cells—tall columnar, pale stained with prominent nucleolus. These cells reach the lumen. Function—support and nutrition, phagocytosis and secretion of hormones.
- Spermatogonia—germ cells, lie near the basal membrane, undergo mitosis to form primary spermatocytes.
- Primary spermatocytes—large cells. Each undergoes meiosis to form two secondary spermatocytes.
- Secondary spermatocytes—smaller, each undergoes meiosis to form two spermatids.
- Spermatids—round cells embedded in apical part of Sertoli cells. Undergoes morphological changes to from spermatozoa by the process of spermiogenesis.
- Spaces between the seminiferous tubules contain loose connective tissue with blood vessels. Also contains interstitial cells of Leydig—round large cells, secrete testosterone—male sex hormones.

56. TESTIS

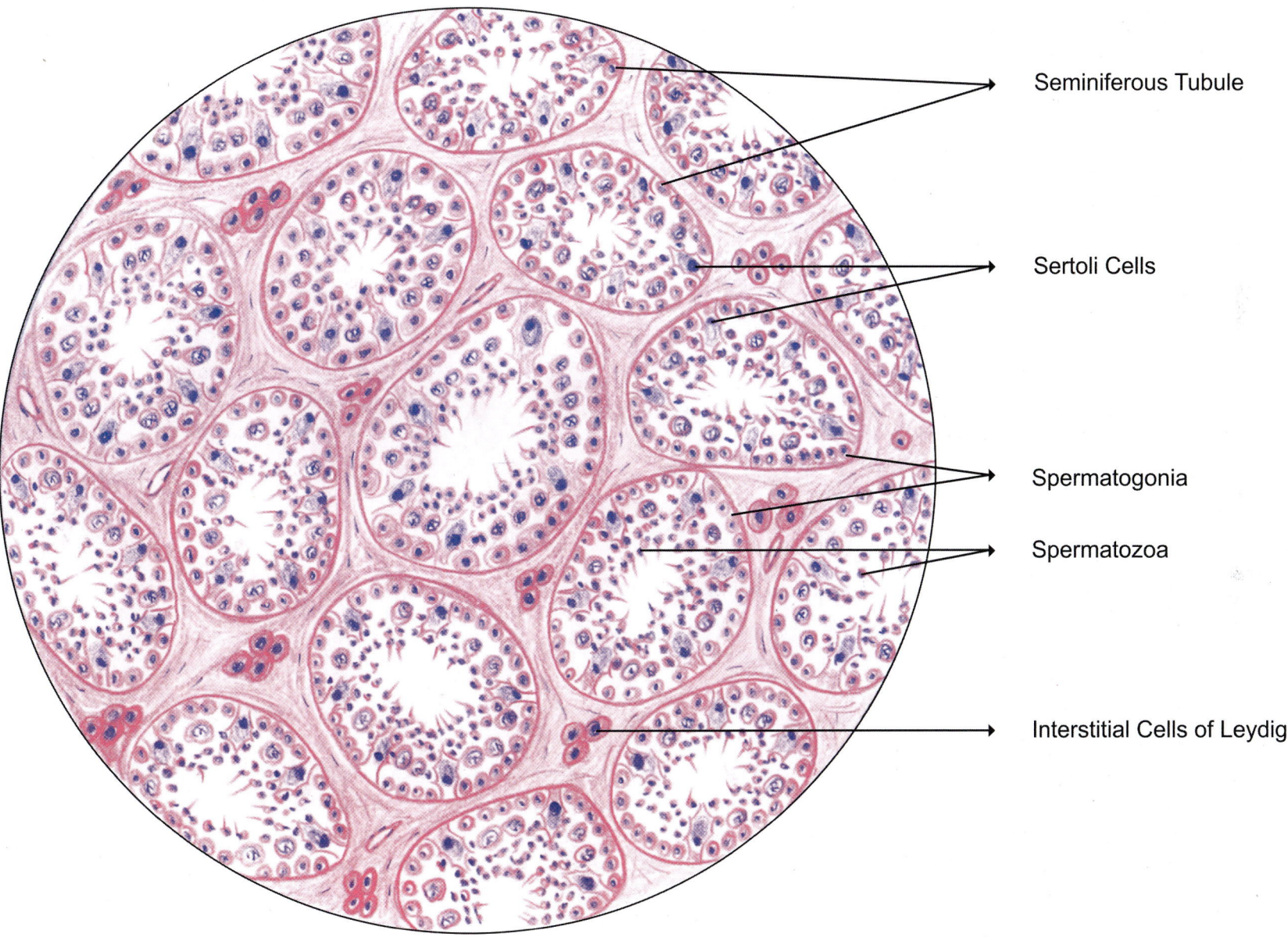

- Seminiferous Tubule
- Sertoli Cells
- Spermatogonia
- Spermatozoa
- Interstitial Cells of Leydig

57. EPIDIDYMIS

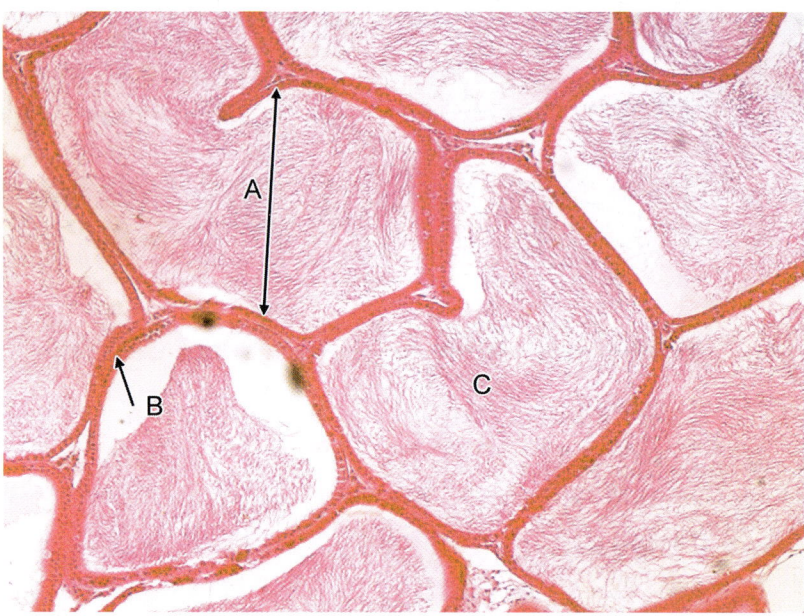

A	Sections of Duct of Epididymis
B	Pseudostratified Columnar Epithelium with Stereocilia
C	Clumps of Spermatozoa

Identification Points

1. **Sections of tubule lined by pseudostratified columnar epithelium with stereocilia.**
2. **Lumen filled with sperms.**
3. **Each tube surrounded by smooth muscle cells.**

- Epididymis is highly coiled single tubular structure.
- Coils of tubules held by fibrous connective tissue.
- Tubule is lined by pseudostratified columnar epithelium with stereocilia. Each tubule is surrounded by smooth muscle cells which help in the transport of spermatozoa through the contraction of tubules.
- Stereocilia are large microvilli for absorption of fluids.
- Function—reabsorb fluid from the testicular secretions.
- Helps in maturation of spermatozoa.

57. EPIDIDYMIS

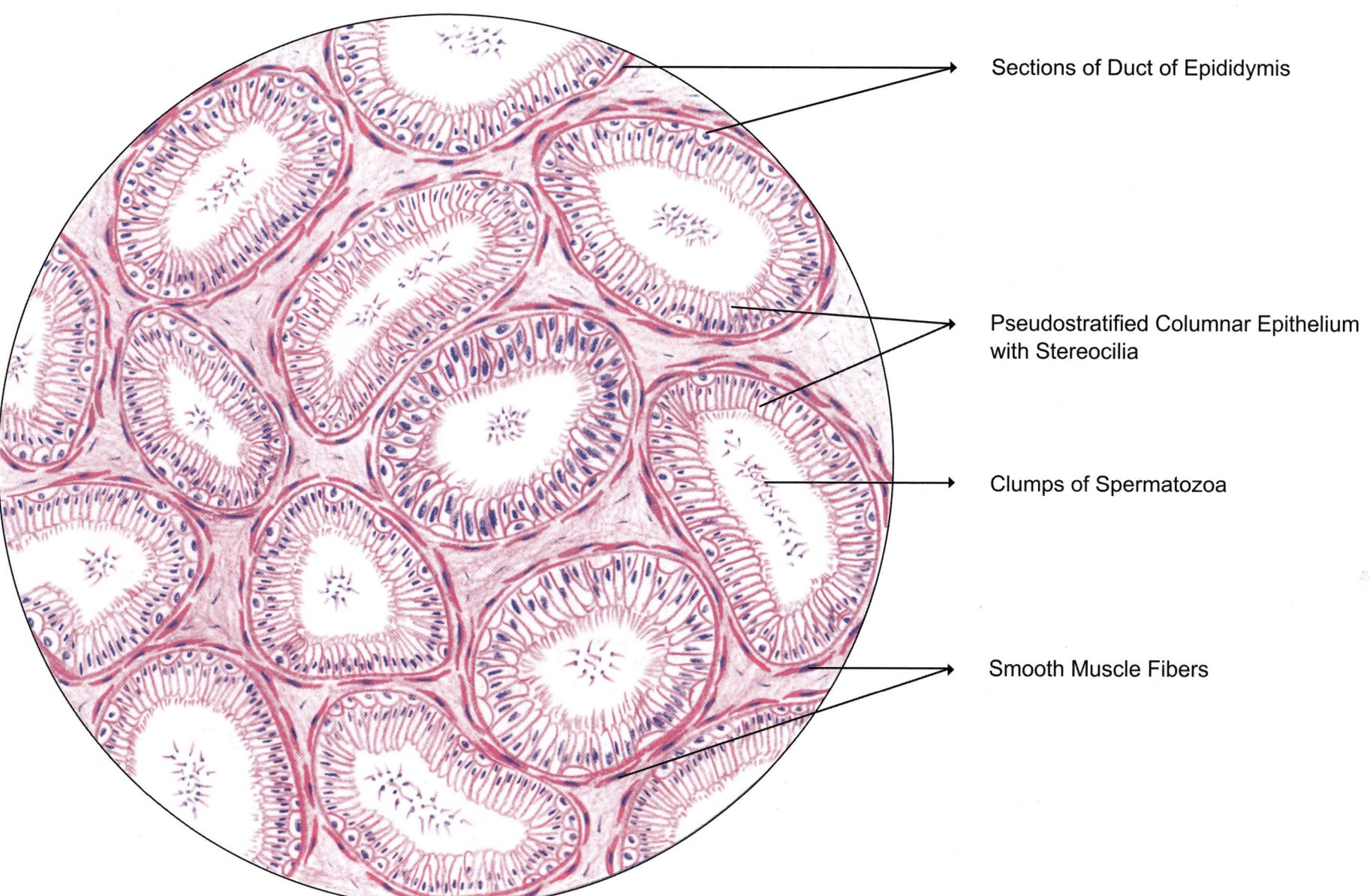

58. DUCTUS DEFERENS/VAS DEFERENS

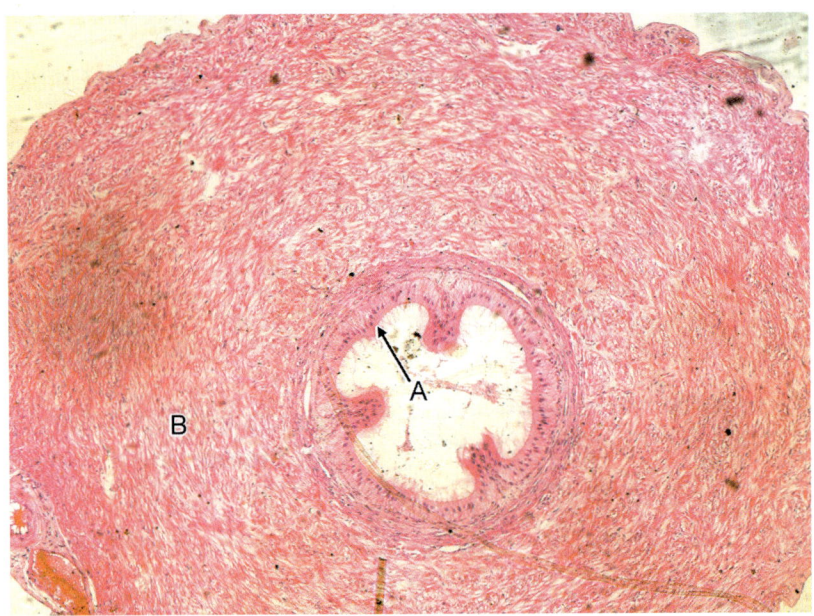

A	Columnar Epithelium
B	Layer of Smooth Muscles

Identification Points

1. **Mucosa lined by simple columnar cells (towards the distal end, it is lined by pseudostratified columnar epilhelium)*.**
2. **Thick muscular tube.**

Also called as vas deferens.

1. Mucous membrane—shows longitudinal folds—lumen is small:
   - Lined by simple columnar cells.
   - Lamina propria—loose connective tissue with elastic fibers.
2. Thick muscle coat—inner circular, outer longitudinal smooth muscles.
3. Outermost layer—adventitia made of connective tissue.
   Function—conveys sperm to the ejaculatory ducts.

---

*Gray's Anatomy, 40th edition. p. 1269.

58. DUCTUS DEFERENS/VAS DEFERENS

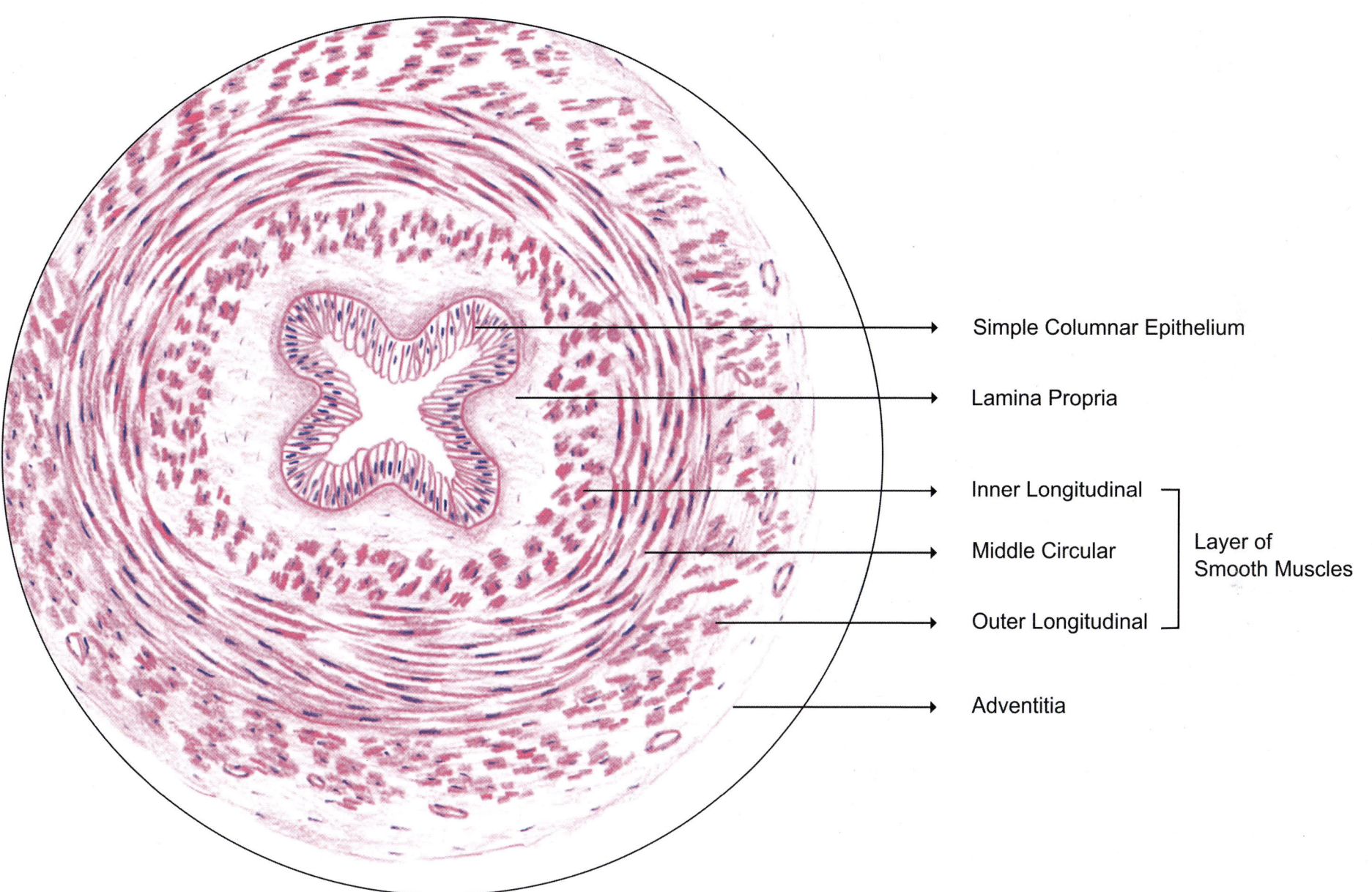

59. PROSTATE

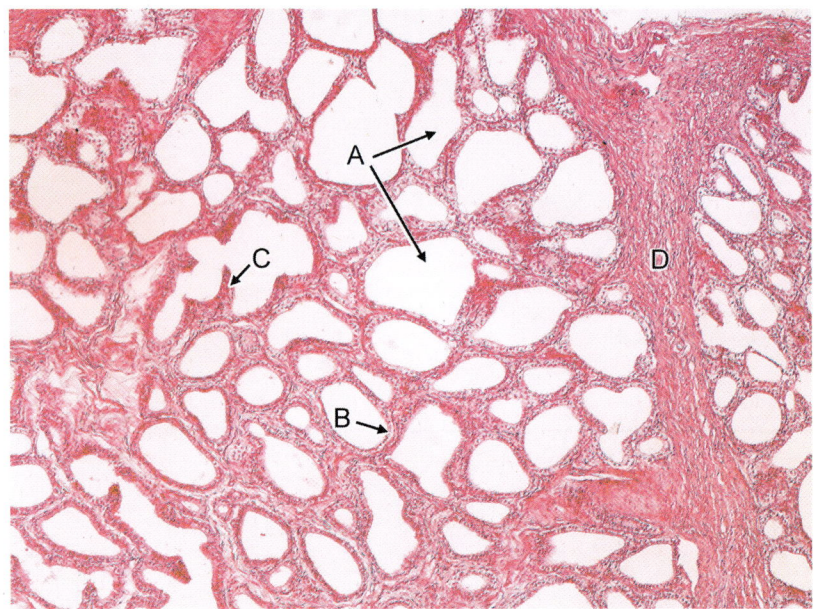

A	Prostatic Glands or Acini
B	Columnar Epithelium
C	Mucosal Folds
D	Fibromuscular Stroma

Identification Points

1. Prostatic glands (acini or follicles) lined by simple columnar epithelium.
2. Mucosa thrown into folds, lumen contains corpora amylacea.
3. Acini separated by thick fibromuscular stroma.

- Tubuloalveolar glands separated by fibromuscular stroma.
- Glands lined by columnar epithelium, mucosa thrown into folds.
- Lumen contains lamellated round masses of corpora amylacea (calcified glycoprotein) which increases with age.
- Fibromuscular stroma—is made of collagen fibers and smooth muscles. It becomes more with age.

59. PROSTATE

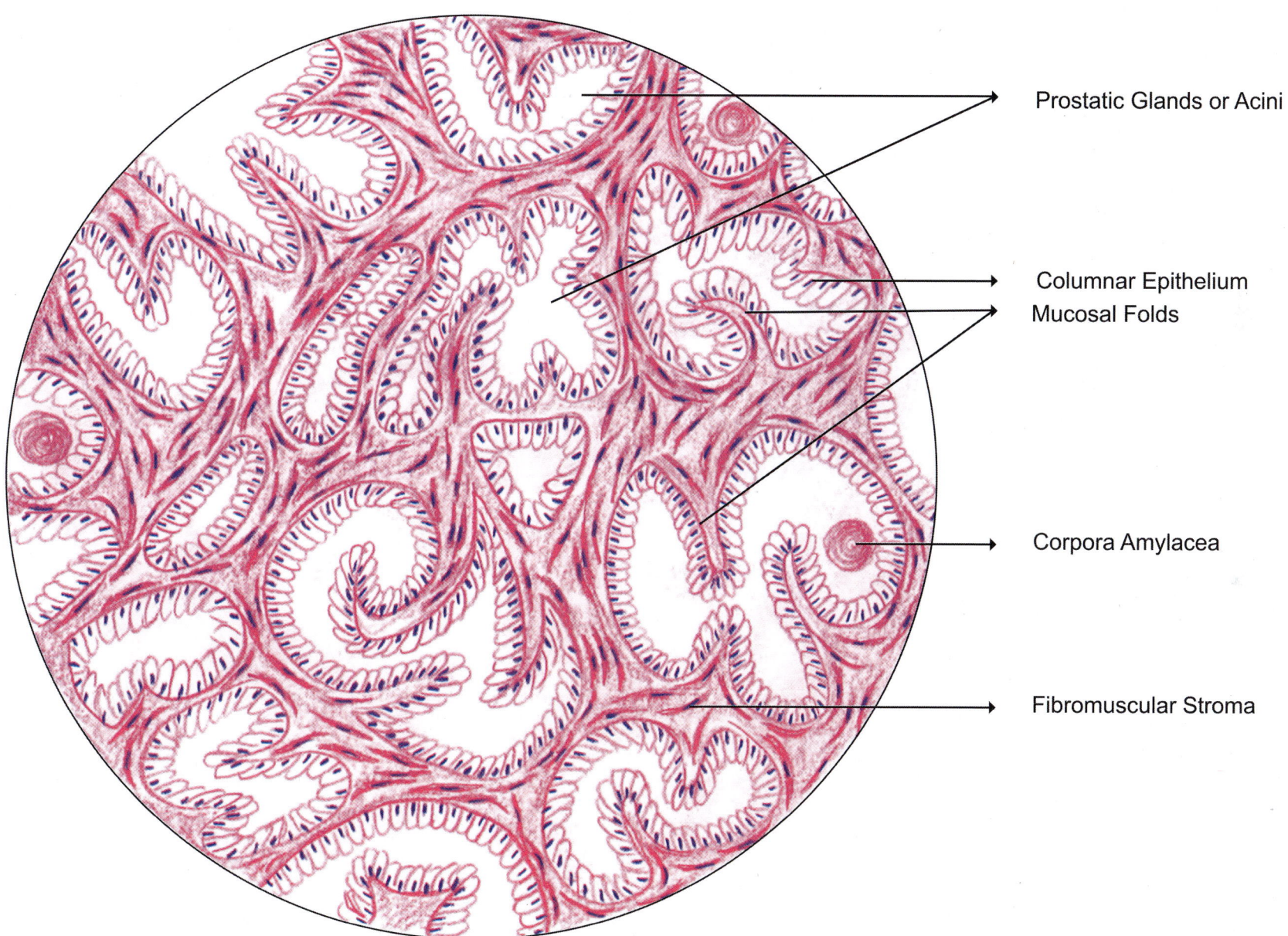

60. SEMINAL VESICLE

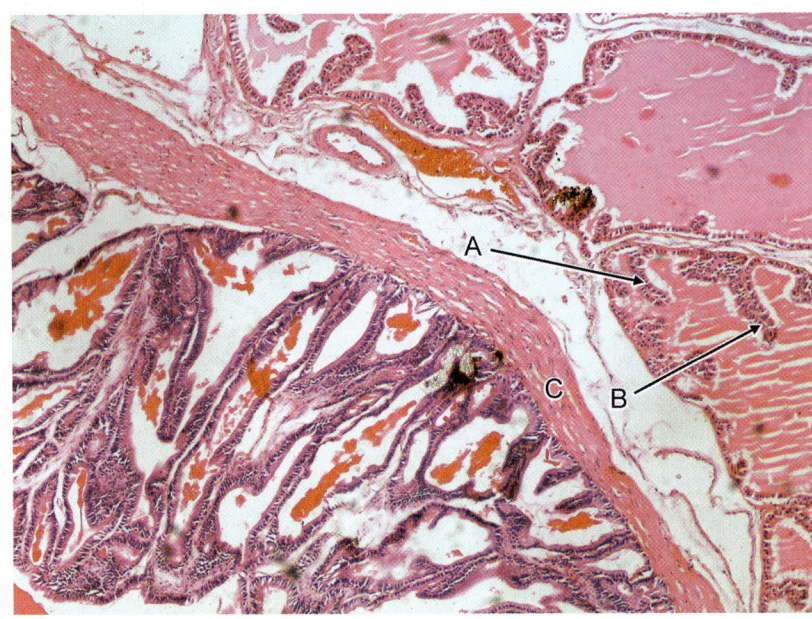

B	Mucosal Folds
C	Smooth Muscle
A	Columnar Epithelium

Identification Points

1. **Lumen is filled with highly convoluted mucosal folds.**
2. **Lining epithelium—pseudostratified columnar type.**

Several sections of tubules seen.
1. Mucosa thrown into folds that branch and anastomose.
   - Lined by simple/pseudostratified columnar cells, goblet cells.
2. Middle layer of smooth muscles.
3. Outer connective tissue covering.

60. SEMINAL VESICLE

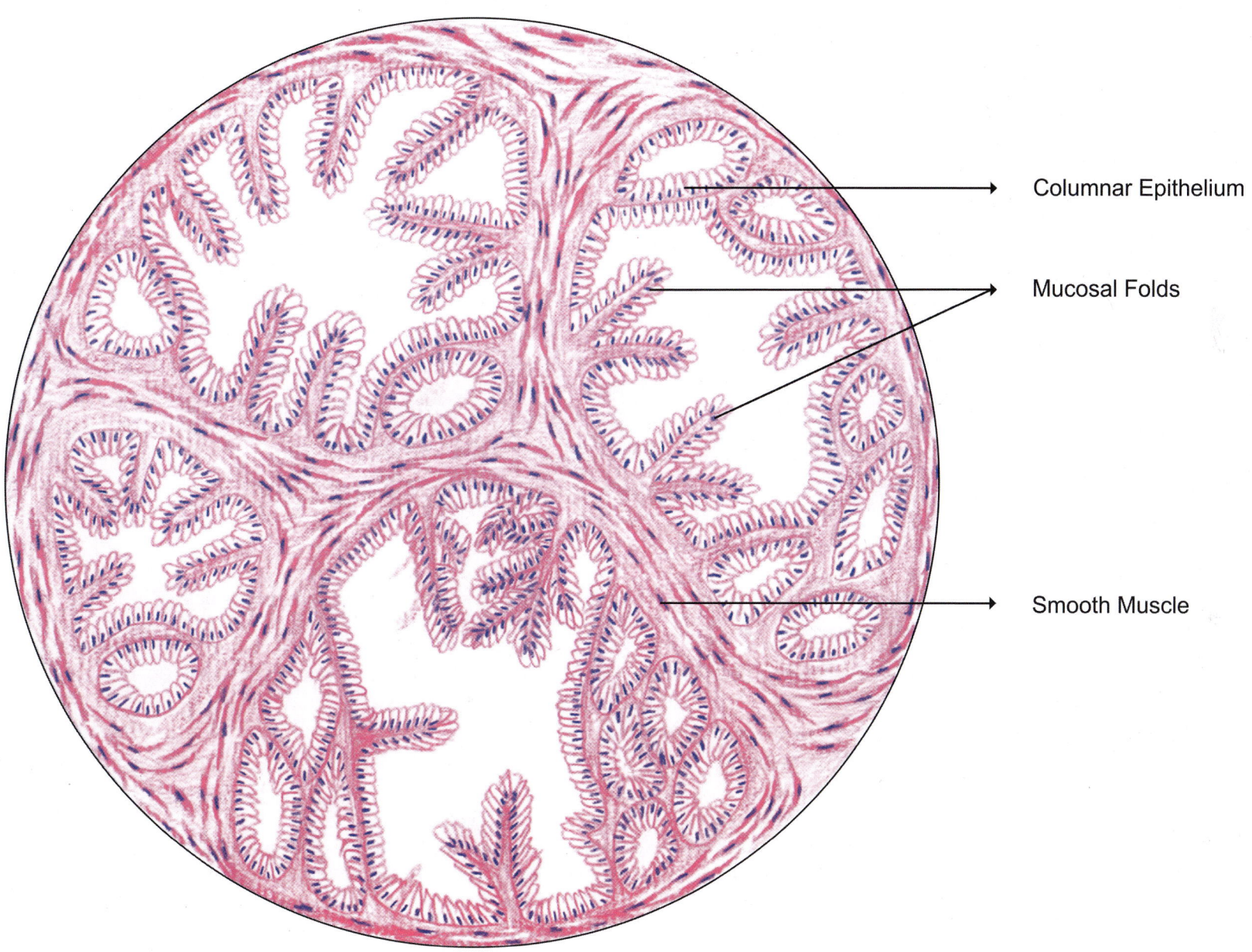

61. OVARY

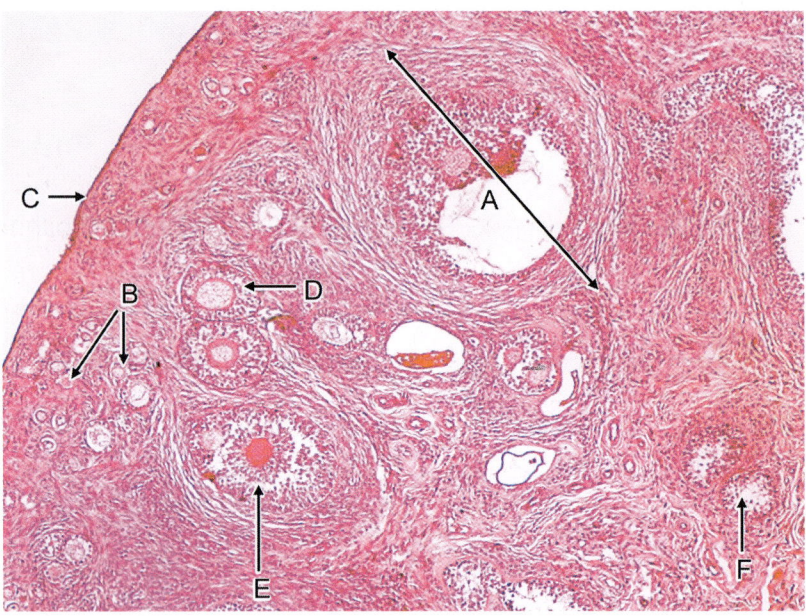

A	Graafian Follicle
B	Primordial Follicle
C	Germinal Epithelium
D	Primary Follicle
E	Secondary Follicle
F	Atretic Follicle

Identification Points

1. **Outer cortex—shows ovarian follicles in different stages of development—primordial, primary, secondary and Graafian follicle.**
2. **Inner medulla—contains connective tissue with blood vessels.**

- Surface lined by germinal epithelium made of cuboidal cells below which lies the connective tissue covering called tunica albuginea.
- Section of ovary divides into outer cortex and inner medulla.
  - Cortex contains follicles in different stages of development separated by the stroma.
  - Primordial follicle—primary oocyte surrounded by flat stromal cells.
  - Primary follicle—primary oocyte surrounded by columnar cells.
  - Secondary follicle—primary oocyte surrounded by several layers of follicular cells with a fluid filled follicular cavity.
  - Graafian follicle-follicular cavity increases in size and oocyte becomes eccentrically located surrounded by cumulus oophoricus. It is attached to wall of follicle by discus proligerus. Surrounding stromal cells form theca interna and fibers form theca externa. Follicular cells and theca interna (thecal glands) secrete estrogen.
  - Corpus luteum—after ovulation the follicular wall becomes collapsed. Follicular cells enlarge, cytoplasm filled with yellow pigment called lutein and secrete progesterone.
- Stroma contains fusiform mesenchyme cells, smooth muscles and reticular fibers.
- Medulla—contains connective tissue with blood vessels and smooth muscles.

61. OVARY

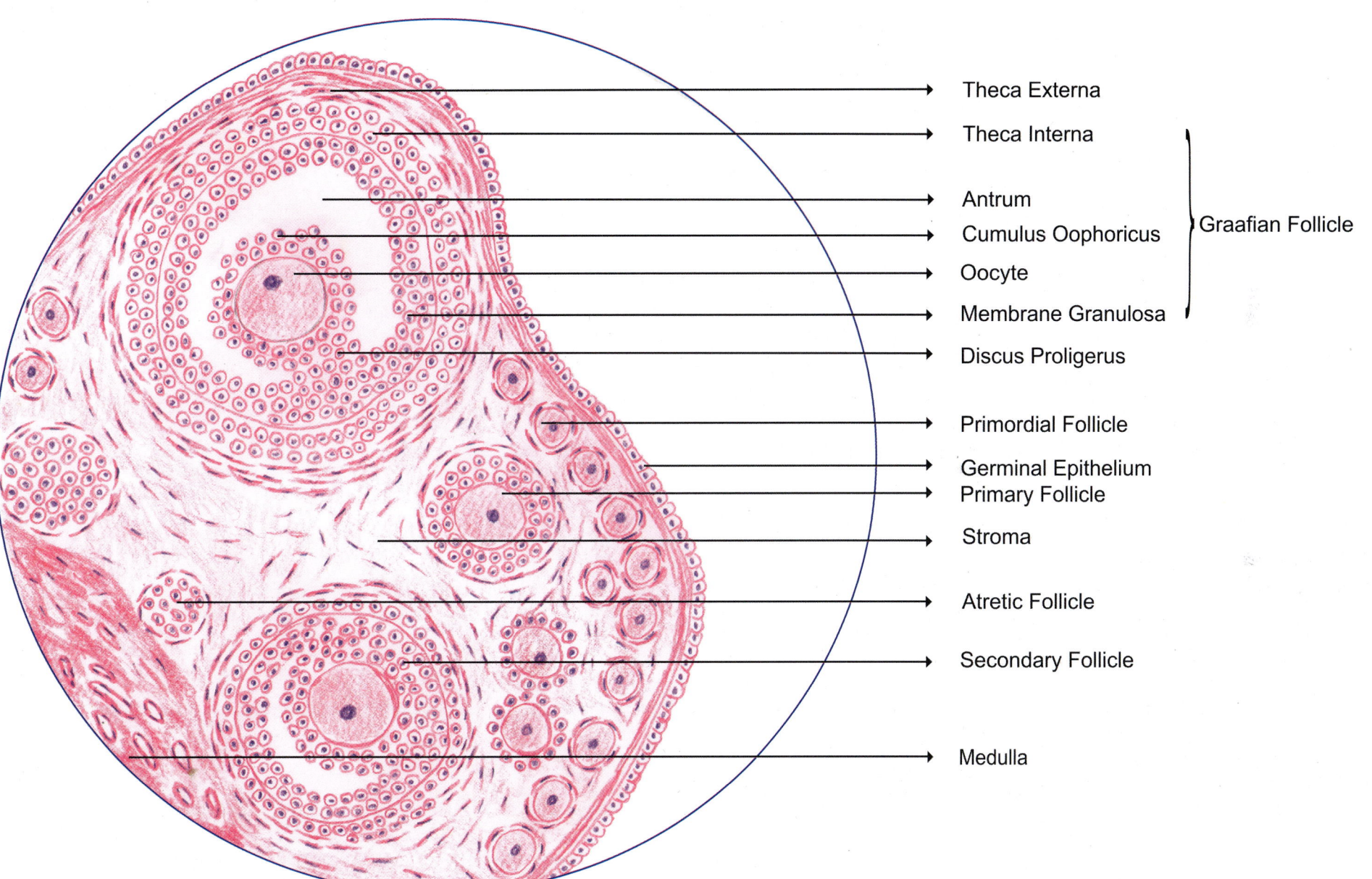

62(A). UTERUS: PROLIFERATIVE

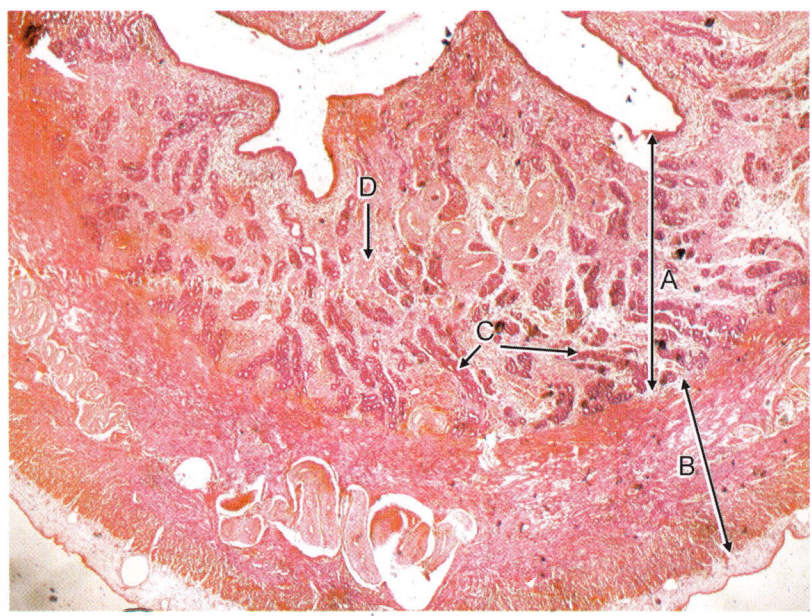

A	Endometrium
B	Myometrium
C	Uterine Glands
D	Spiral Arteries

Identification Points

1. **Inner endometrium—lined by simple columnar cells. Stroma contains tubular uterine glands and spiral arteries.**
2. **Middle thick muscular layer—myometrium.**
3. **Outer perimetrium.**

It has three layers—outer perimetrium, middle myometrium and inner endometrium.
- Endometrium—lined by columnar epithelium. Stroma is highly cellular contains simple tubular glands and spiral arteries. Endometrium is divided into:
  - Outer pars (stratum) functionalis which is shed during the menstrual phase.
  - Inner pars (stratum) basalis which helps in regeneration of the shed endometrium.
- Depending on the phase of menstrual cycle, the endometrium shows cyclical changes:
  - Proliferative phase—under the influence of estrogen the endometrium increases in thickness, glands elongate, spiral arteries reach up to the surface and stromal cells increases in number.
  - Secretory phase—under the influence of progesterone, the endometrium further increases in thickness. Glands are dilated and tortuous giving a saw-toothed appearance in sections. Spiral arteries further coil upon themselves.
- Myometrium—three ill-defined layers of smooth muscles. Blood vessels run inbetween the muscles fibers forming living ligatures.
- Perimetrium—made of connective tissue covering.

62(A). UTERUS: PROLIFERATIVE

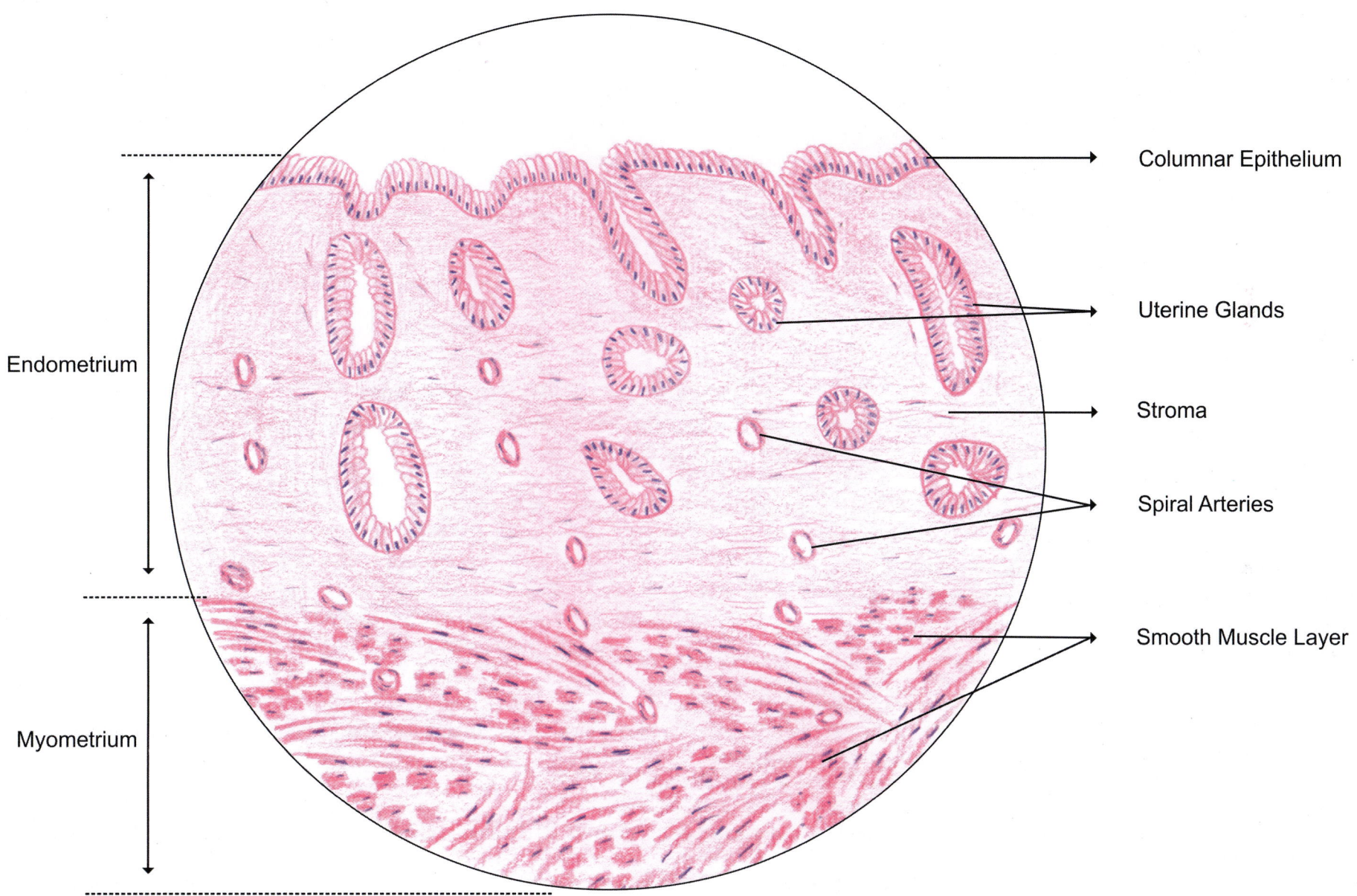

62(B). UTERUS: SECRETORY

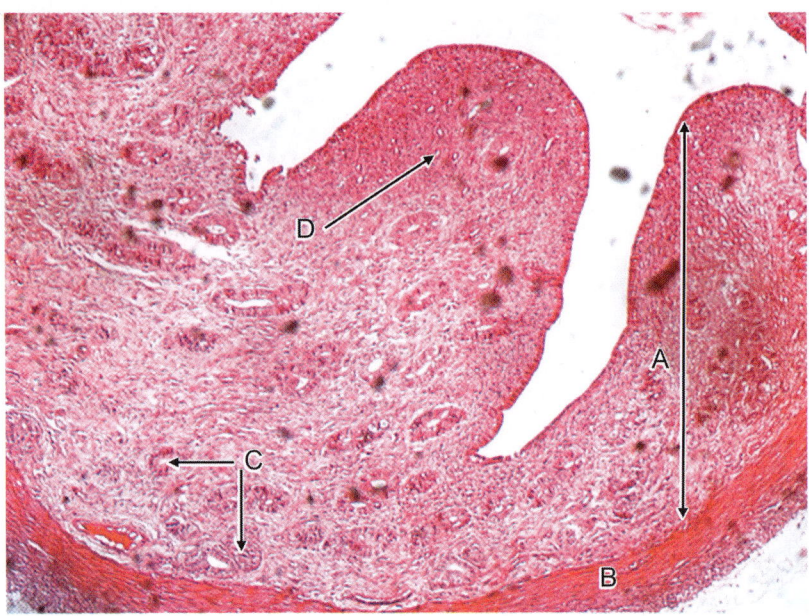

A	Endometrium
B	Myometrium
D	Spiral Arteries
C	Tortuous Uterine Glands

Identification Points

1. **Inner endometrium—lined by simple columnar cells. Stroma contains tubular uterine glands and spiral arteries.**
2. **Middle thick muscular layer—myometrium.**
3. **Outer perimetrium.**

It has three layers—outer perimetrium, middle myometrium and inner endometrium.
- Endometrium—lined by columnar epithelium. Stroma is highly cellular contains simple tubular glands and spiral arteries. Endometrium is divided into:
  - Outer pars (stratum) functionalis which is shed during the menstrual phase.
  - Inner pars (stratum) basalis which helps in regeneration of the shed endometrium.
- Depending on the phase of menstrual cycle, the endometrium shows cyclical changes:
  - Proliferative phase—under the influence of estrogen the endometrium increases in thickness, glands elongate, spiral arteries reach up to the surface and stromal cells increases in number.
  - Secretory phase—under the influence of progesterone, the endometrium further increases in thickness. Glands are dilated and tortuous giving a saw-tooth appearance in sections. Spiral arteries further coil upon themselves.
- Myometrium—three ill-defined layers of smooth muscles. Blood vessels run inbetween the muscles fibers forming living ligatures.
- Perimetrium—made of connective tissue covering.

62(B). UTERUS: SECRETORY

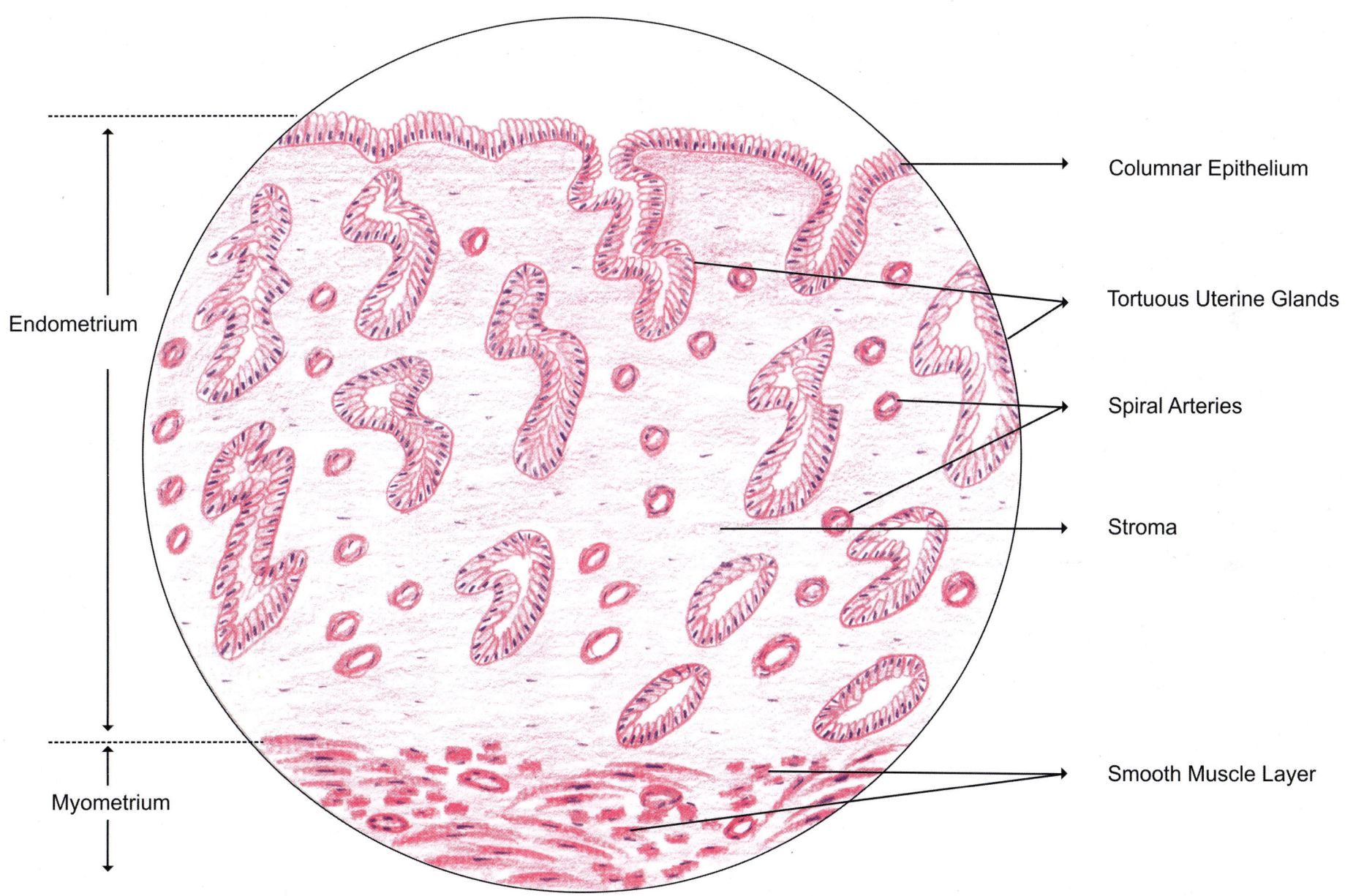

63. FALLOPIAN TUBE

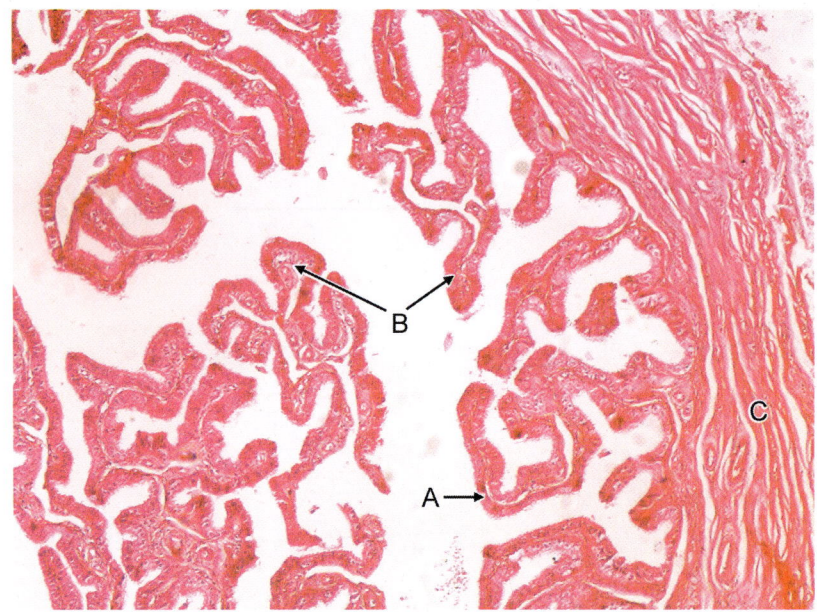

A	Simple Ciliated Columnar Epithelium
B	Mucosal Folds
C	Layer of Smooth Muscles

Identification Points

1. **Lining epithelium—simple columnar cells with cilia.**
   Mucosa thrown into folds filling the lumen.
2. **Muscular tube.**

1. Mucus layer—thrown into numerous branching and anastomosing folds which almost fill the lumen. Lined by columnar cells—cells are of two types:
   – Ciliated cells—which help in movement of ova towards the uterine cavity.
   – Non-ciliated cells—secretory or peg cells, secretions help in nourishment of ova.
2. Muscle layer—inner circular and outer longitudinal layer of smooth muscles.
3. Serosa—lined by flat squamous cells of peritoneum.

63. FALLOPIAN TUBE

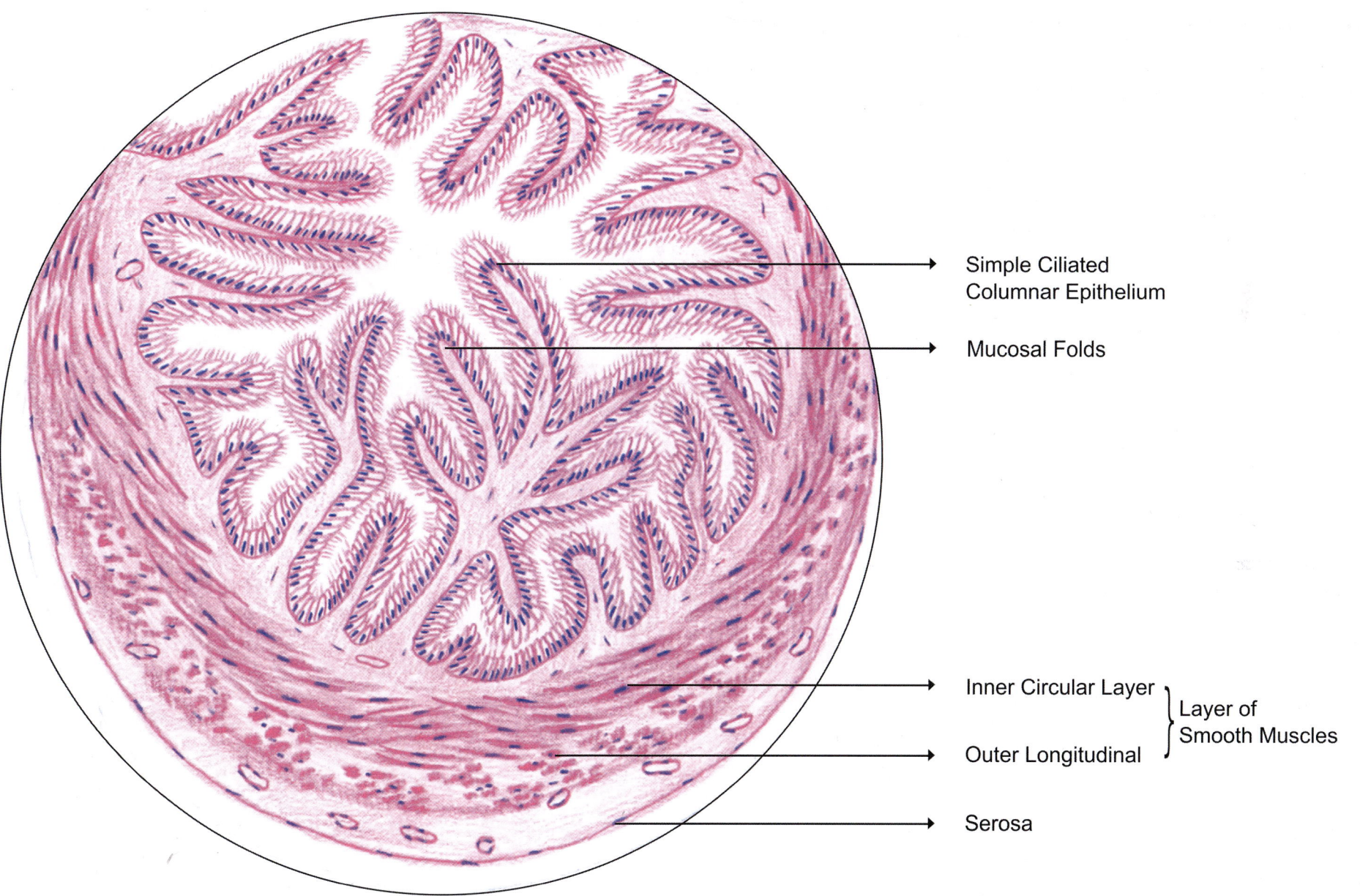

64(A). MAMMARY GLAND: INACTIVE STAGE

Mammary Gland—Inactive Stage

1. More of connective tissue with fat cells.
2. Indistinct alveoli, duct, lobules and lobes.

64(A). MAMMARY GLAND: INACTIVE STAGE

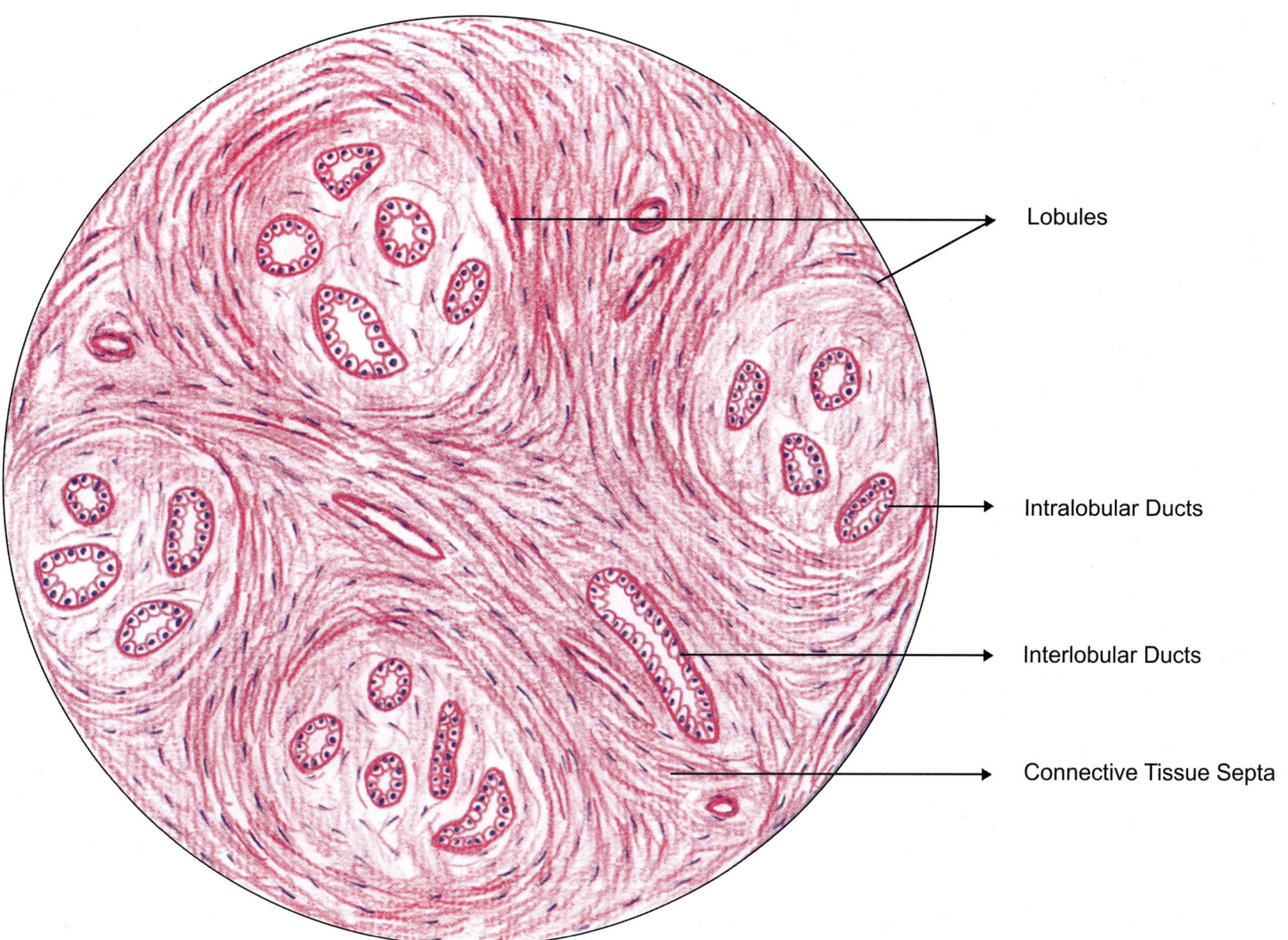

- Lobules
- Intralobular Ducts
- Interlobular Ducts
- Connective Tissue Septa

64(B). MAMMARY GLAND: IN PREGNANCY

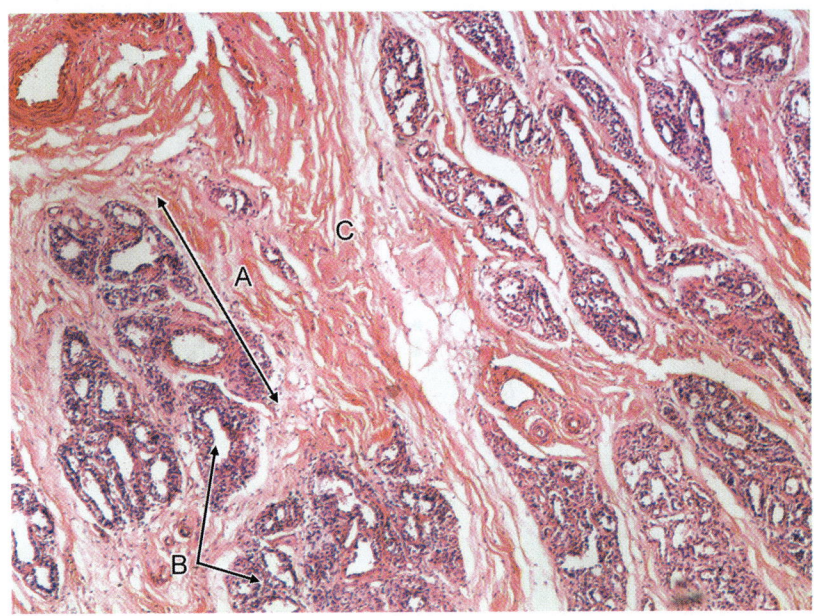

A	Lobules
B	Alveoli
C	Connective Tissue Septa

Mammary Gland—in Pregnancy

1. Well-developed lobes, lobules and duct system.
2. Alveoli present but empty.
3. Connective tissue and fat cells comparatively less.

64(B). MAMMARY GLAND: IN PREGNANCY

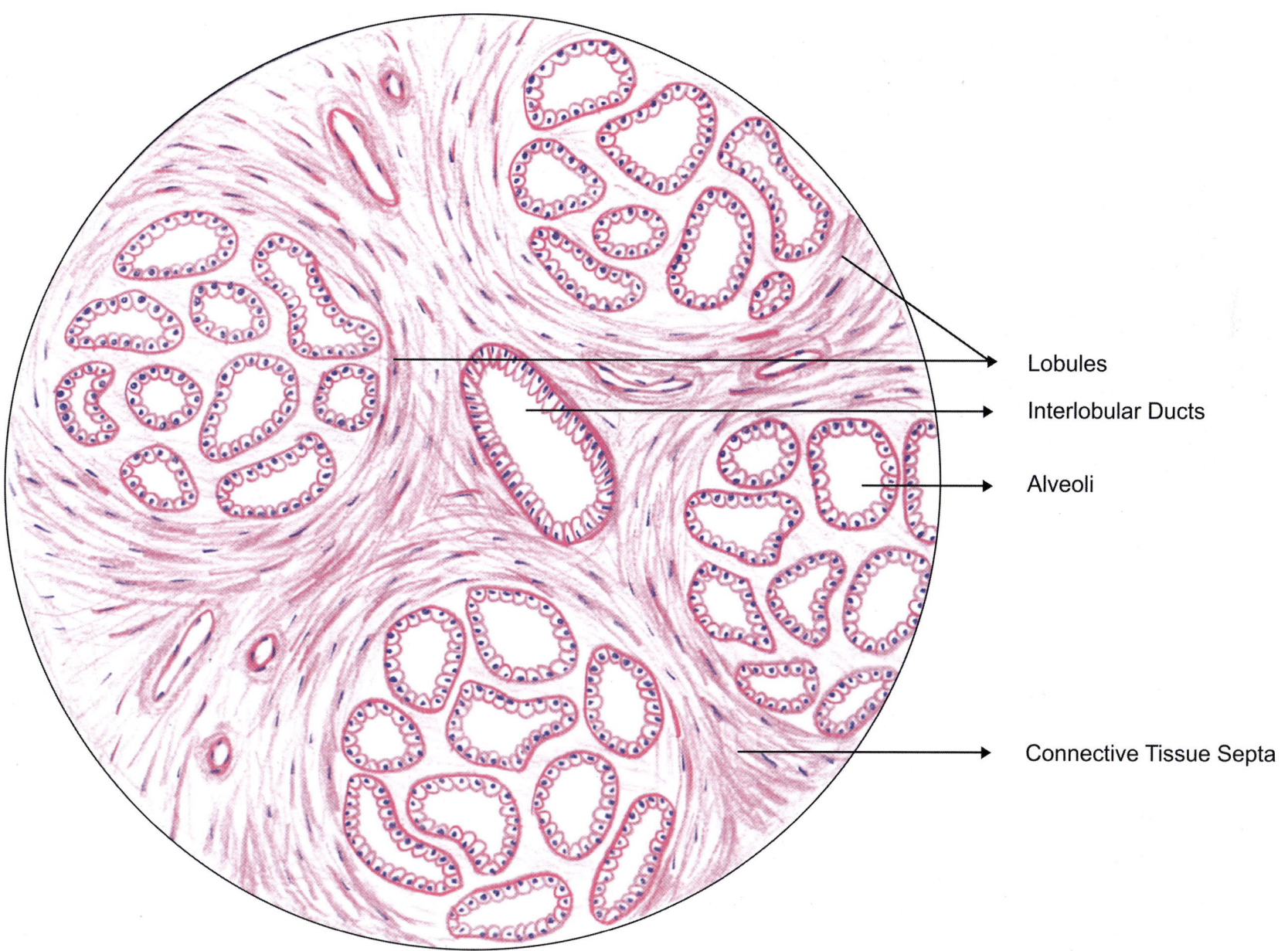

64(C). MAMMARY GLAND: IN LACTATION

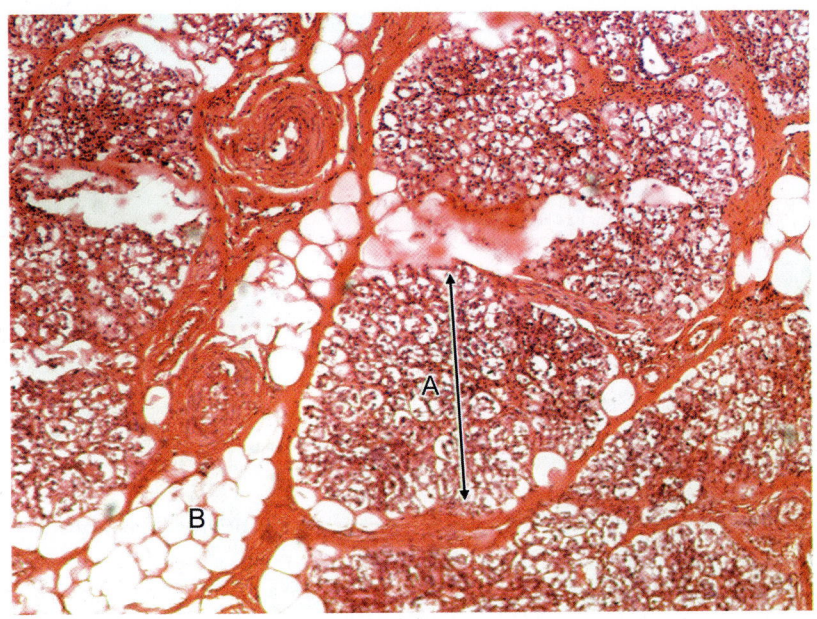

A	Alveoli with Secretions
B	Adipose Tissue

Mammary Gland—in Lactation

1. Alveoli of various size and shape, filled with secretion.
2. Well-developed ducts.
3. Connective tissue stroma separating into lobes and lobules.

64(C). MAMMARY GLAND: IN LACTATION

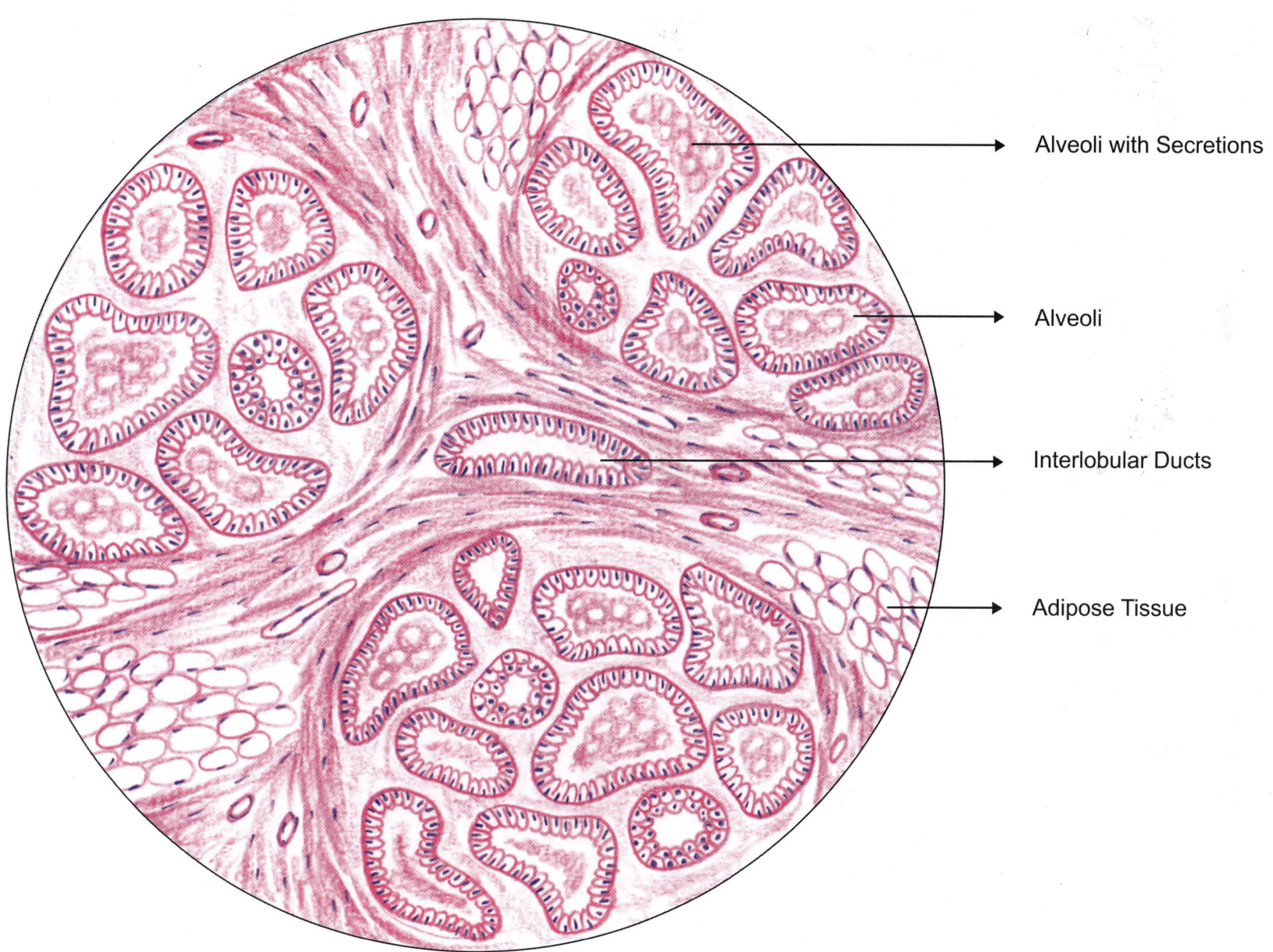

- Alveoli with Secretions
- Alveoli
- Interlobular Ducts
- Adipose Tissue

65. UMBILICAL CORD

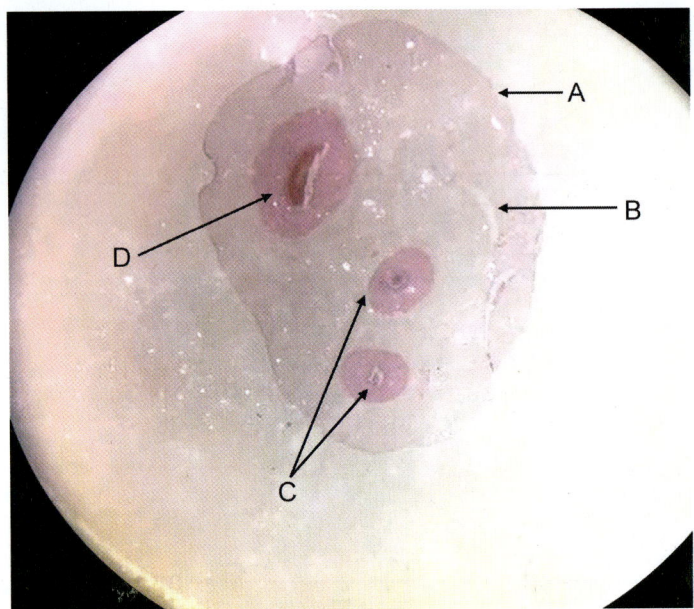

A	Amnion
B	Wharton's Jelly
C	Umbilical Arteries
D	Umbilical Vein

Identification Points

1. Two muscular arteries and one vein seen.
2. Wharton's jelly (embryonic mesenchyme) surrounding the vessels with outer amniotic covering.

- Cut section shows outer layer of amniotic membrane made of flattened squamous cells.
- Mucoid embryonic connective tissue known as Wharton's jelly surrounds the blood vessels.
- It contains two umbilical arteries and one umbilical vein.
- Two muscular arteries right and left from fetus carry the deoxygenated blood to placenta.
- Only one vein is seen (left vein is left, right has obliterated) which carries oxygenated blood from placenta to fetus.
- Length of the cord is 50 cm, with diameter of 2 cm.

65. UMBILICAL CORD

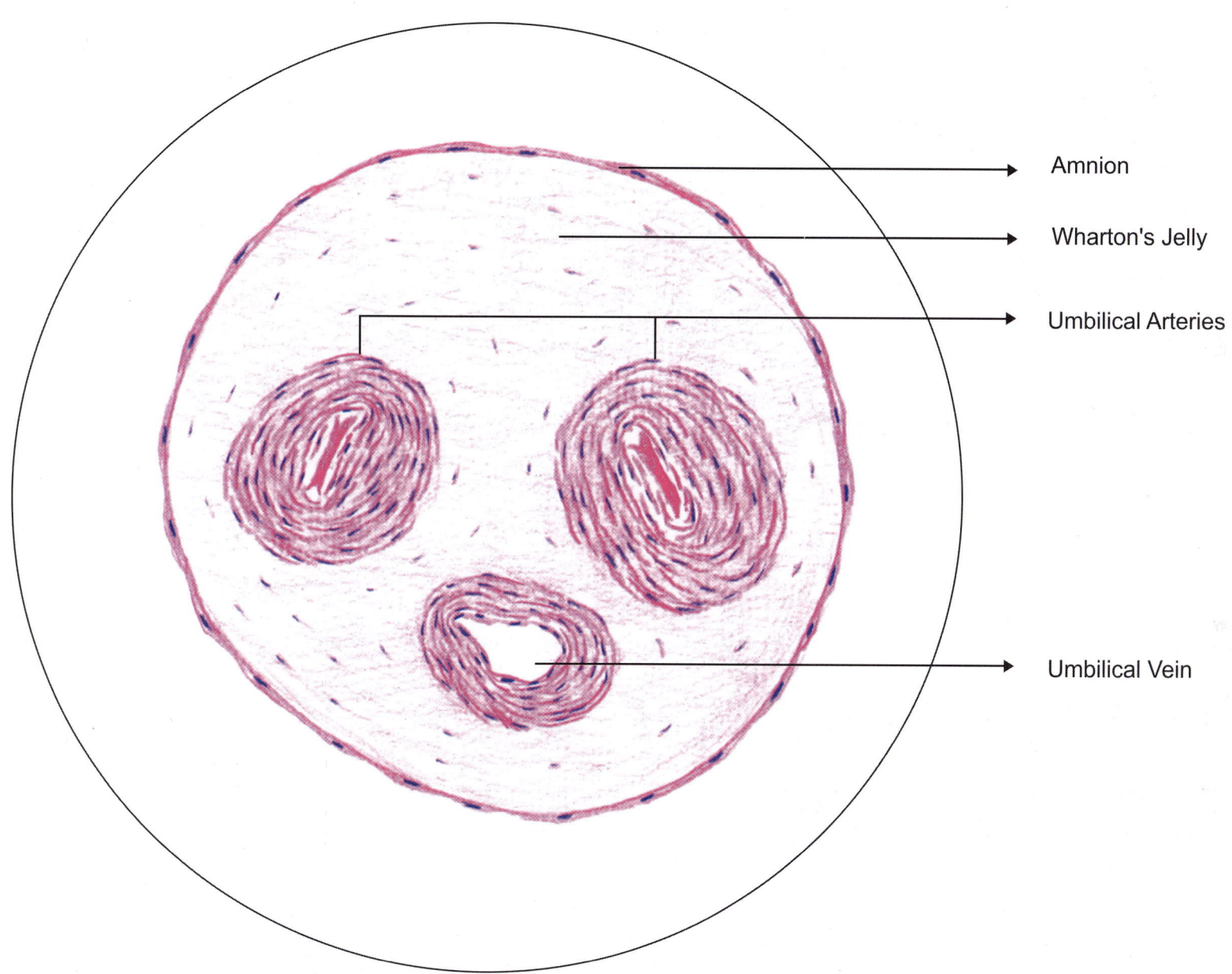

66. PLACENTA

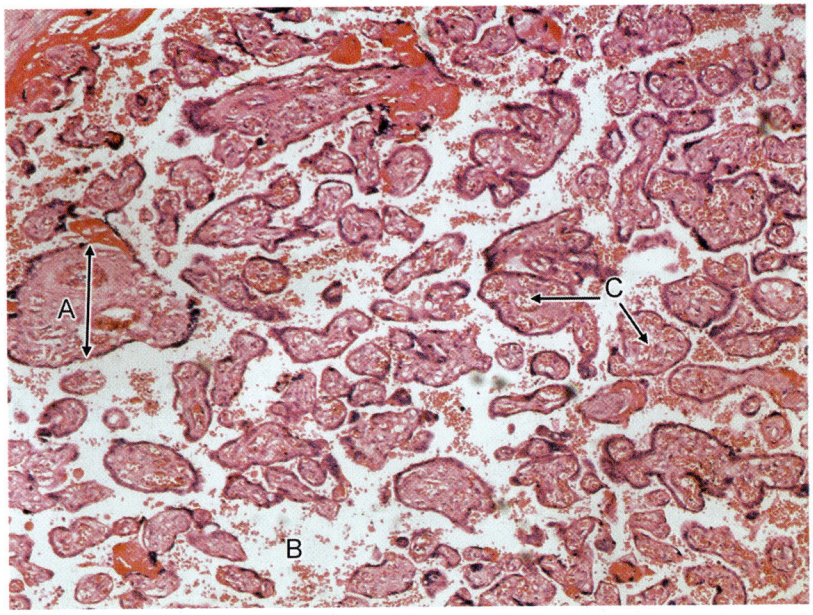

A	Chorionic Villus
B	Intervillous Space
C	Fetal Vessels

Identification Points

1. Sections of chorionic villi seen.
2. Villi with embryonic connective tissue core containing fetal capillaries and surrounded by outer syncytiotrophoblasts and inner cytotrophoblasts.

- Chorionic villi form a part of placenta and are involved in exchange of materials between mother and fetus. Chorionic villi sections appear in different shapes and sizes. Chorionic villi are described as primary, secondary and tertiary during development.
- Chorionic villi:
  – Have a lining of outer syncytiotrophoblasts and inner cytotrophoblasts. Cytotrophoblasts cells are pale staining with well-defined cell boundaries whereas syncytiotrophoblasts are dark staining without a cell boundary, forming a syncytium.
  – In full-term placenta chorionic villi have only outer syncytiotrophoblasts lining.
- Central core is made of embryonic connective tissue with fetal capillaries.
- Intervillous space contains maternal blood cells.
- Function of placenta—nutrition to fetus, excretion of waste products, respiration, protection and hormone production.
- Placental barrier—membrane across which exchange takes place. It consists of syncytiotrophoblast, cytotrophoblast, connective tissue and endothelium of fetal capillaries.

66. PLACENTA

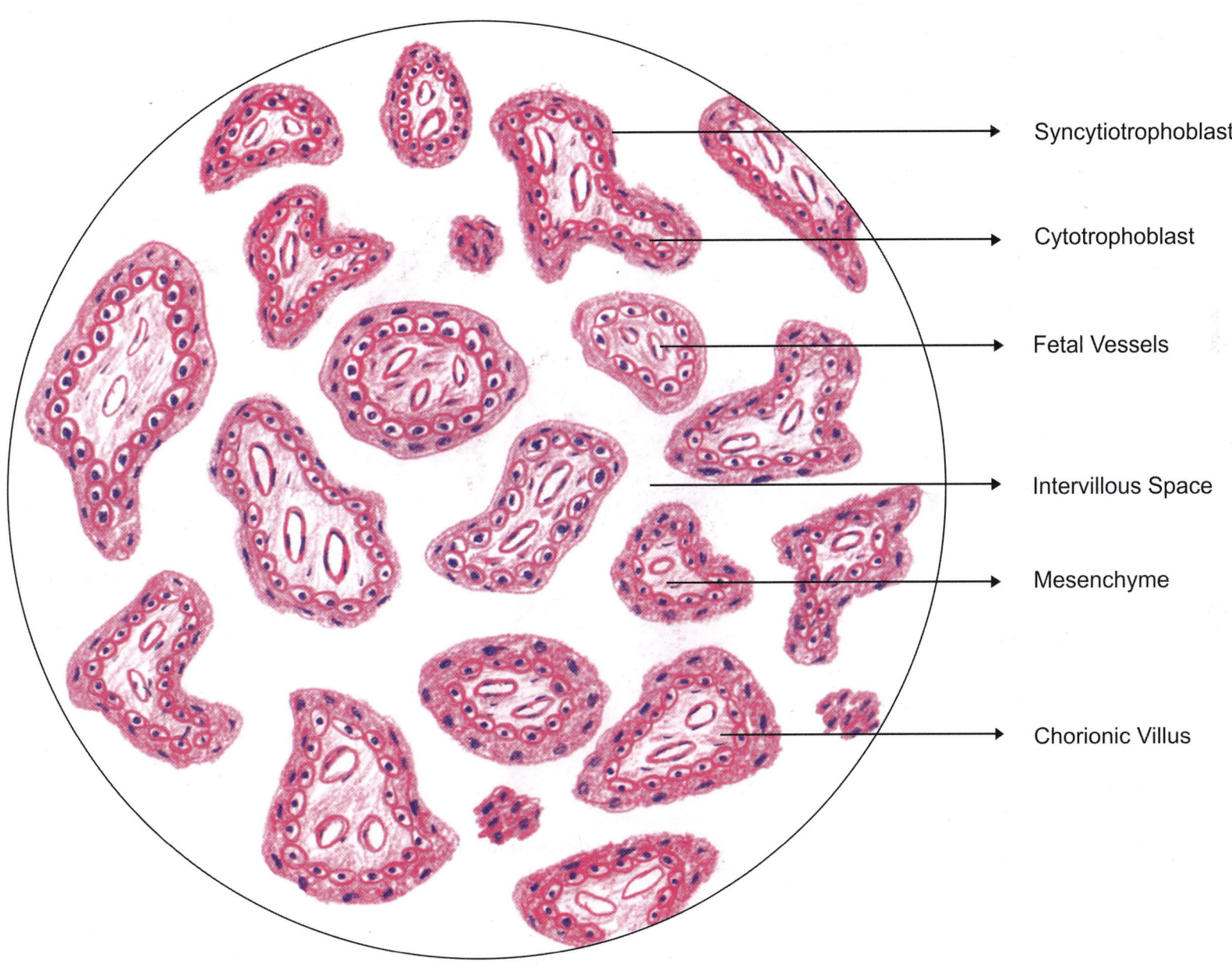

67. PITUITARY GLAND

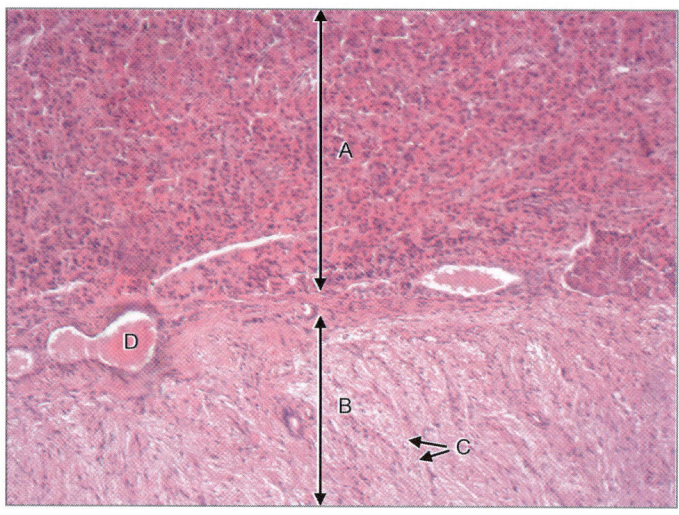

A	Pars Anterior
B	Nerve Fibers in Pars Posterior
C	Pituicytes
D	Colloid Follicles in Pars Intermedia

Identification Points

1. **Adenohypophysis with chromophobes and chromophils arranged in groups.**
2. **Neurohypophysis with nerve fibers and pituicytes.**

- It has two parts—adenohypophysis and neurohypophysis.
- Adenohypophysis/pars anterior—made of clusters of cells separated by sinusoids.
    - Two cell types—chromophobes and chromophils
        » Chromophobes do not take up stain and appear pale.
        » Chromophils have granules in their cytoplasm. Depending on the staining two types:
            - Acidophils which take up acidic stain and appear eosinophilic.
            - Basophils which take up basic stain and appear basophilic.
    - Pars intermedia has colloid filled vesicles.
- Neurohypophysis/pars posterior
    - Made of unmyelinated nerve fibers, cell bodies of which are located in the paraventricular and supraoptic nuclei of hypothalamus.
    - Terminal parts of axons are called Herring bodies which contain the hormones produced by the hypothalamus.
    - Supporting cells called pituicytes are present in between the nerve fibers.
- Hormones produced:
    - Acidophils: Somatotrophs—growth hormone; mammotrophs—prolactin. Basophils: Corticotrophs—adrenocorticotropic hormone; thyrotrophs—thyroid stimulating hormone; gonadotrophs—follicle stimulating hormone and luteinizing hormone (female)/interstitial cell stimulating hormone (male).
    - Pars intermedia—melanocytes stimulating hormone.
    - Pars posterior—stores vasopressin/antidiuretic hormone and oxytocin.

67. PITUITARY GLAND

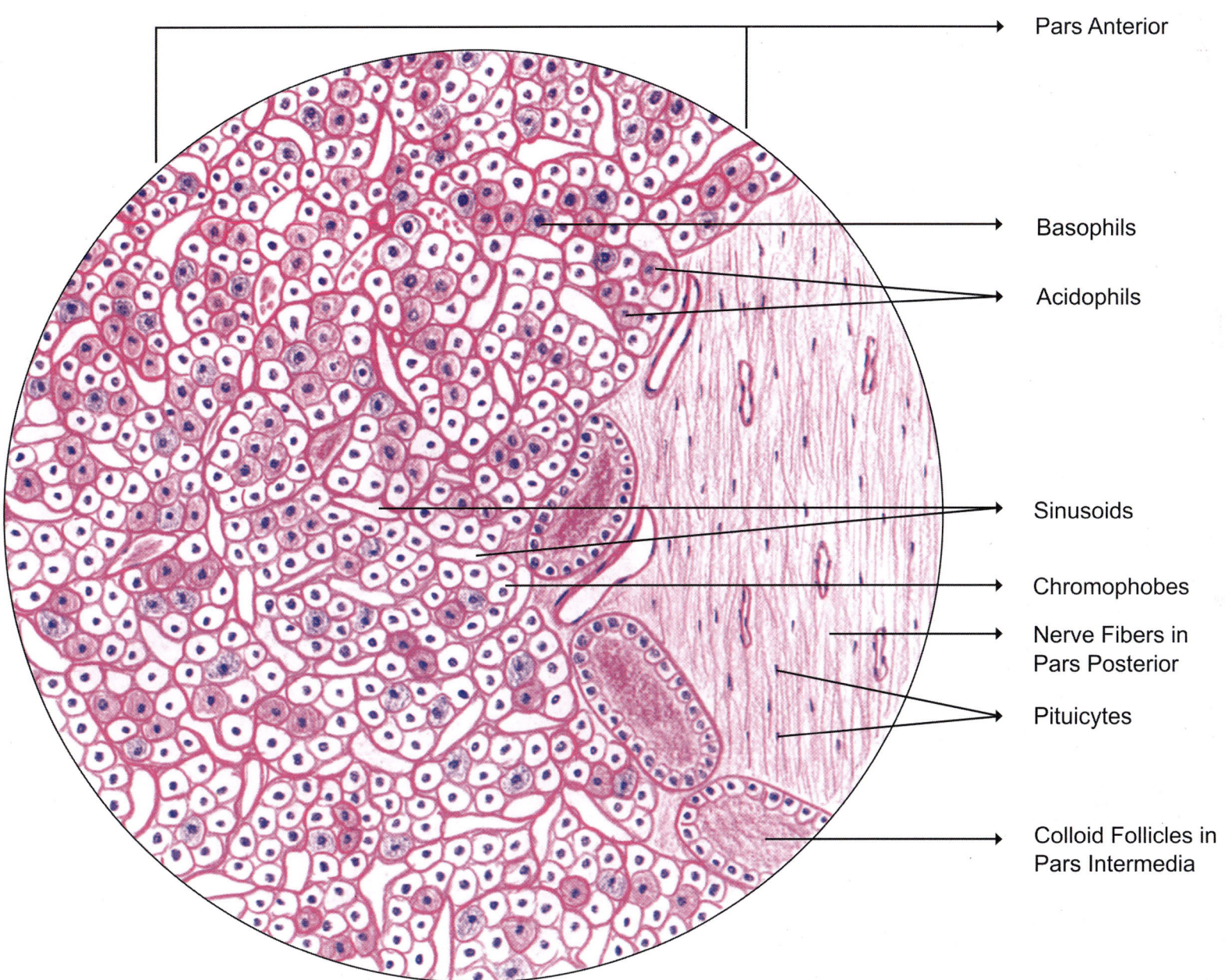

68. SUPRARENAL/ADRENAL GLAND

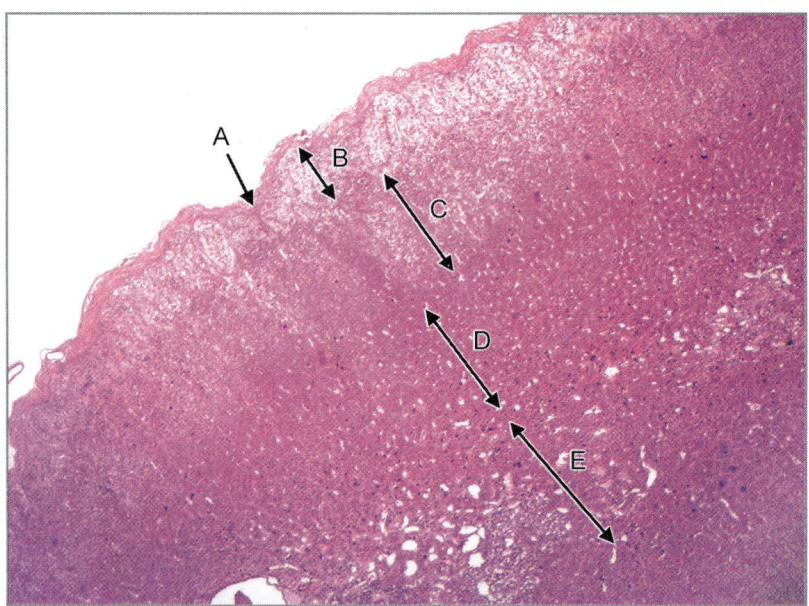

A	Capsule
B	Zona Glomerulosa
C	Zona Fasciculata
D	Zona Reticularis
E	Chromaffin Cells in Medulla

Identification Points

1. **Cortex and medulla differentiated.**
2. **Cortex with outer zona glomerulosa, middle zona fasciculata and inner zona reticularis.**
3. **Medulla with polyhedral chromaffin cells in groups.**

- Connective tissue capsule surrounds the gland. Divided into outer cortex and inner medulla.
- Cortex—three layers depending on arrangement of cells:
    1. Zona glomerulosa—outermost layer, outer 1/5th. Polyhedral cells arranged in the form of inverted U-shape.
    2. Zona fasciculata—middle 3/5th. Polyhedral cells are arranged in the form of straight columns separated by sinusoids. Cells contain lipids which give a spongy appearance to cells.
    3. Zona reticularis—inner 1/5th. Cells arranged in the form of network of branching and anastomosing cords, separated by capillaries.
- Medulla—large chromaffin cells in groups separated by sinusoids.
- Hormones produced:
    – Zona glomerulosa—mineralocorticoid called aldosterone—for electrolyte and water balance.
    – Zona fasciculata—glucocorticoids called cortisone and cortisol—for carbohydrate and protein metabolism.
    – Zona reticularis—sex hormones—estrogen and androgens.
    – Medulla—catecholamine—adrenaline and nor adrenaline.

68. SUPRARENAL/ADRENAL GLAND

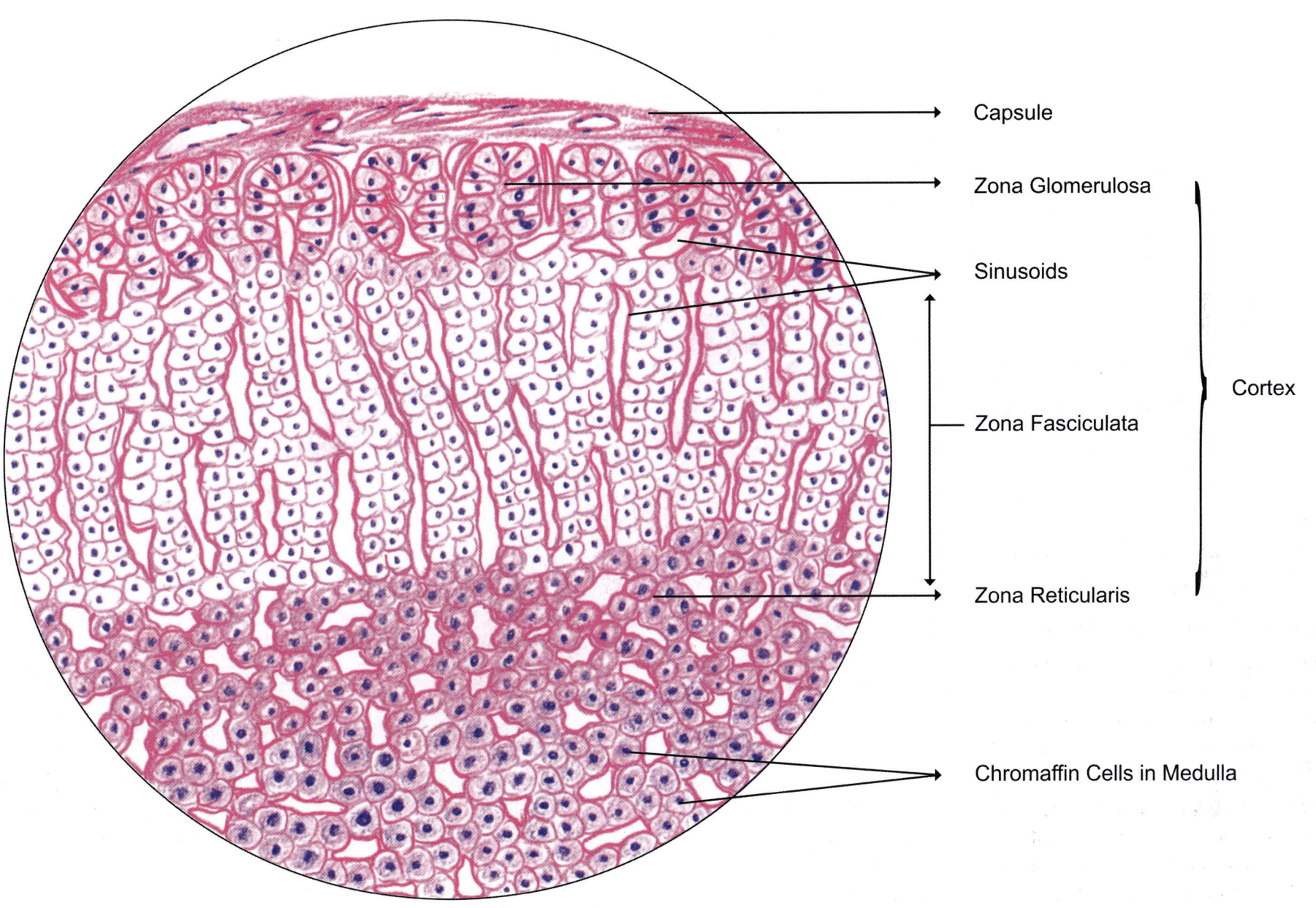

69. THYROID AND PARATHYROID

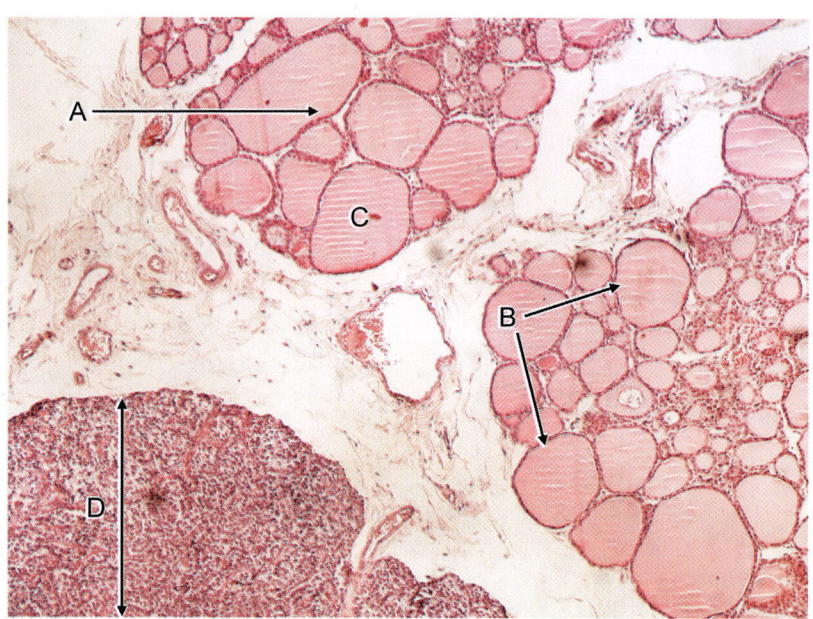

A	Thyroid
B	Follicles Lined by Cuboidal Cells
C	Colloid
D	Parathyroid

Identification Points

1. **Sections of follicles of various sizes filled with colloid, lined by cuboidal cells.**
2. **Parafollicular cells present.**
3. **Highly vascular tissue—plenty of capillaries seen.**

- Fibrous capsule surrounds the gland, sends septa inside dividing the gland into lobules. Each lobule contains follicles of various sizes separated by connective tissue containing numerous capillaries.
- Follicles are filled with eosinophilic homogenous material called colloid (iodinated thyroglobulin).
- Follicle lined by follicular cells resting on a basement membrane. Cells vary in shape depending on the activity of the gland normally they are cuboidal in shape.
  - When inactive, the cells are flat squamous type with abundant colloid.
  - When highly active, the cells are columnar with scanty colloid.
- Parafollicular cells or C cells are located between the follicular cells and basement membrane or in between the follicles—pale staining with eccentric nuclei.
- Hormones produced:
  - Follicular cells secrete tri-iodothyronine (T3) and tetra-iodothyronine (T4/ thyroxin). T3 is more active than T4. These hormones influence the metabolic rate of cells.
  - Parafollicular cells secrete thyrocalcitonin which regulates calcium metabolism by lowering the blood calcium levels.
- Parathyroid gland:
  - Connective tissue capsule send septa which divide the gland into lobules.
  - Each lobule contains cords/clusters of cells separated by numerous sinusoids.
- Two types of cells:
  1. Chief cells or principal cells—more numerous, small round cells with clear cytoplasm.
  2. Oxyphil cells—few in number, large cells with eosinophilic cytoplasm. Appear at the time of puberty.
- Hormones produced:
  - Chief cells produce parathyroid hormone (parathormone)—which increase the blood calcium levels.
  - Oxyphil cells—function not known.

69. THYROID AND PARATHYROID

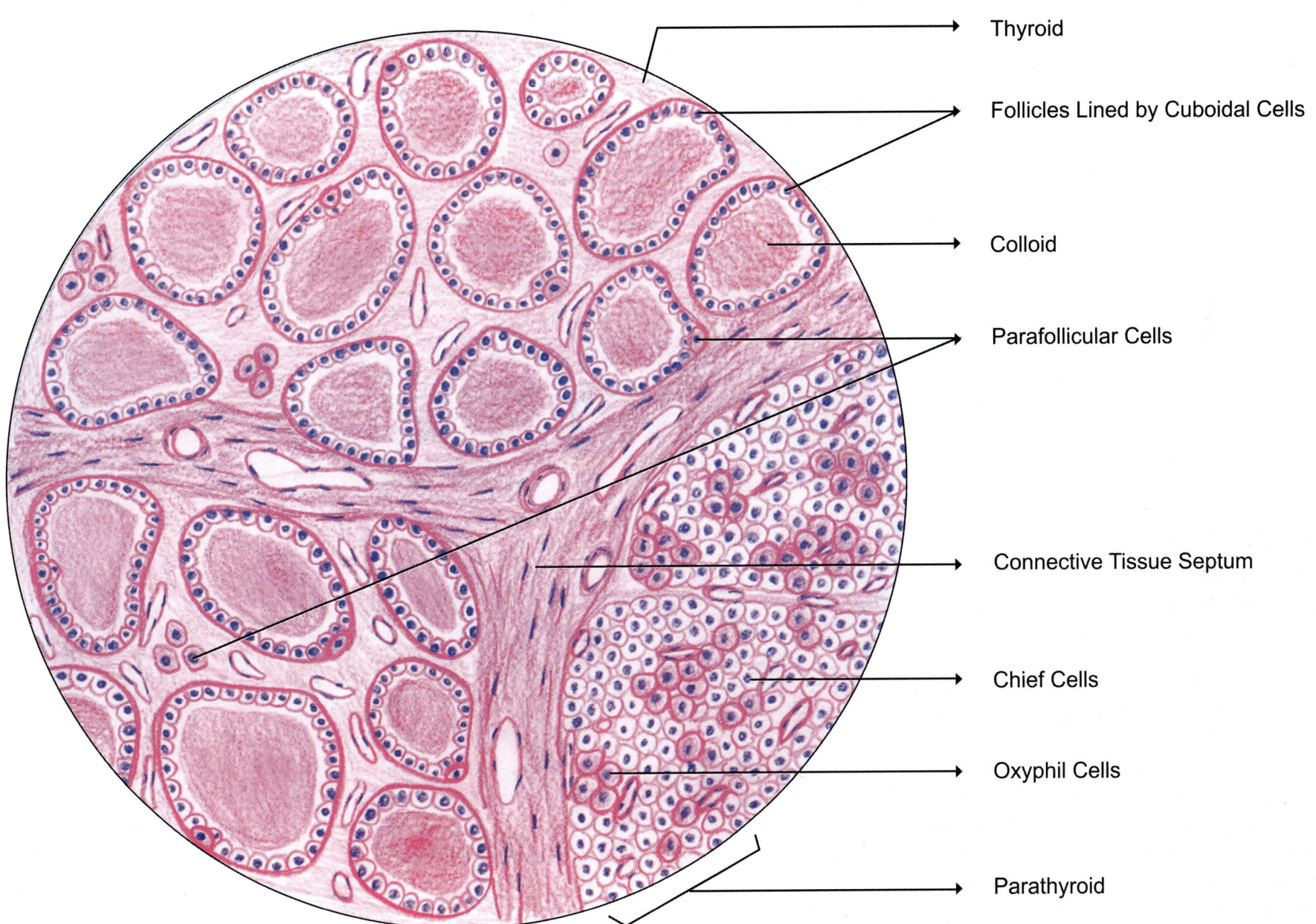

70. CORNEA

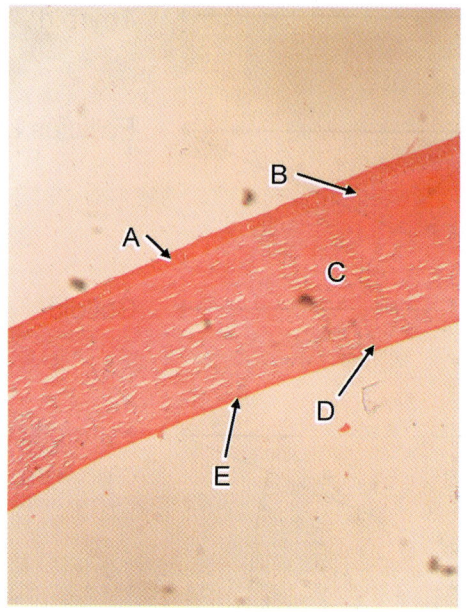

A	Stratified Squamous Non-keratinized Epithelium
B	Bowman's Membrane
C	Substantia Propria
D	Descemet's Membrane
E	Simple Squamous Endothelium

Identification Points

1. **Five layered structure.**
2. **Outer stratified squamous epithelium—non-keratinized.**
3. **Middle thick layer of substantia propria.**

- Anterior 1/6th of tunica externa of wall of the eyeball.
- Cornea is transparent, avascular and richly innervated.
- Five layers of cornea are:
    1. Anterior epithelium—outermost layer, non-keratinized stratified squamous epithelium 4–5 layers thick.
    2. Bowman's membrane (anterior limiting membrane)—is the thickened basement membrane of anterior epithelium.
    3. Substantia propria—thickest layer consists of several layers of collagen fibers with fibroblasts.
    4. Descemet's membrane (posterior limiting membrane)—is the basement membrane of posterior epithelium.
    5. Posterior epithelium—inner layer, simple squamous endothelium.
- Regular arrangement of collagen fibers in substantia propria and avascularity makes cornea transparent.
- Rich nerve supply.
- Nutrition of cornea: Outer layers from—tear film, inner layers—aqueous humor.

70. CORNEA

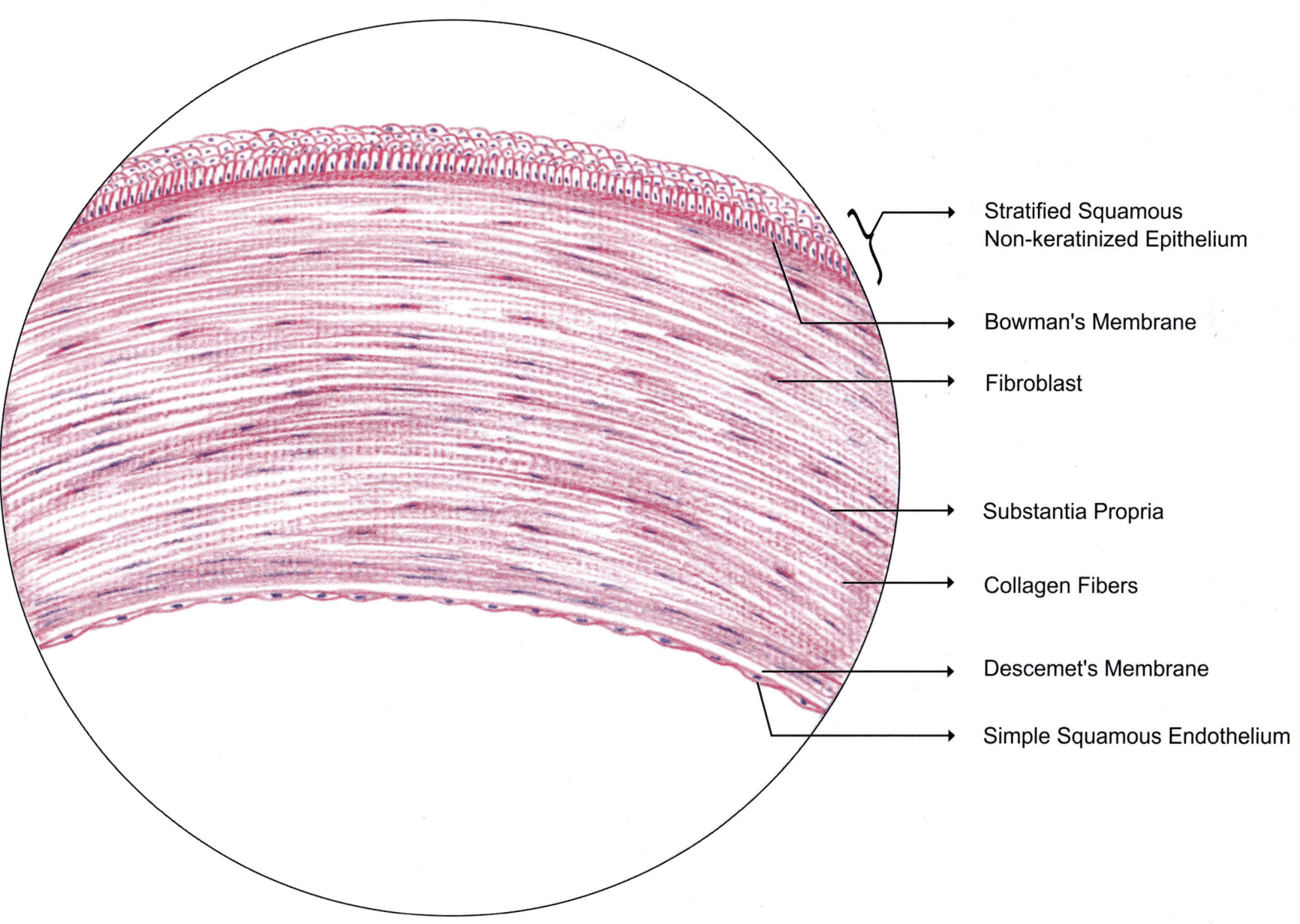

71. CORNEOSCLERAL JUNCTION

SCLEROCORNEAL JUNCTION OR LIMBUS

- At limbus corneal epithelium continues with conjunctival epithelium.
- Bowman's layer ends at the limbus.
- Corneal stroma continues with substantia propria of sclera.
  - Stroma of the sclera is different from that of cornea. In sclera, the collagen fibers of stroma are randomly arranged which makes it opaque, whereas in cornea, they are regularly arranged making it transparent.
  - Sclera is thinner than the cornea.
  - At this junction, canal of Schlemm is present. It is lined by flat endothelial cells. It drains the aqueous humor from anterior chamber into episcleral veins.
- Medial to the canal of Schlemm, the Descemet's membrane continues as trabecular meshwork.
- Sclera is made of three layers:
  1. Episcleral layer—outer covering of loose connective tissue beneath the bulbar conjunctiva.
  2. Substantia propria—layer of irregularly arranged collagen fibers.
  3. Suprachoroidal lamina—inner most layer of delicate fibrous connective tissue.

71. CORNEOSCLERAL JUNCTION

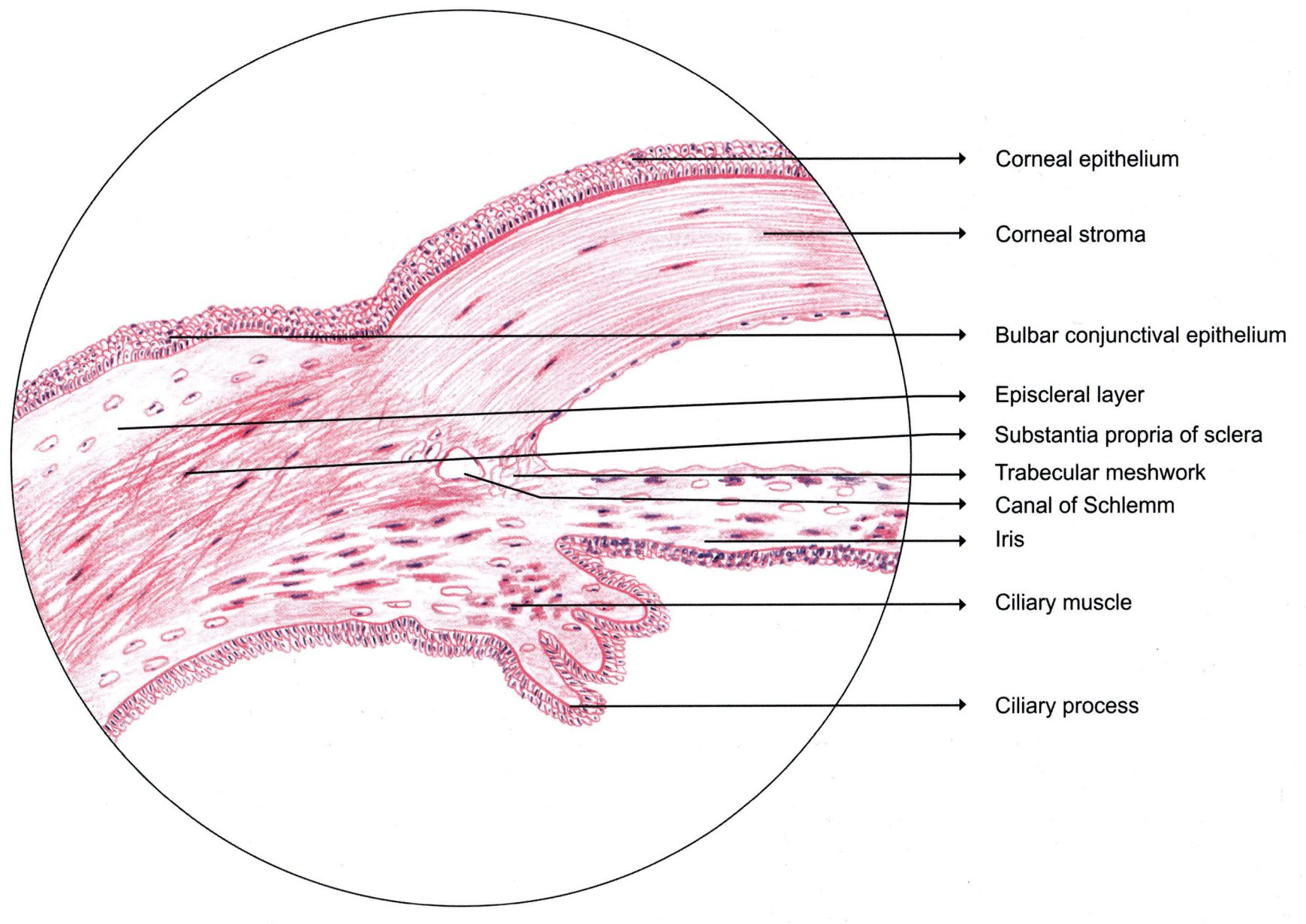

72. RETINA

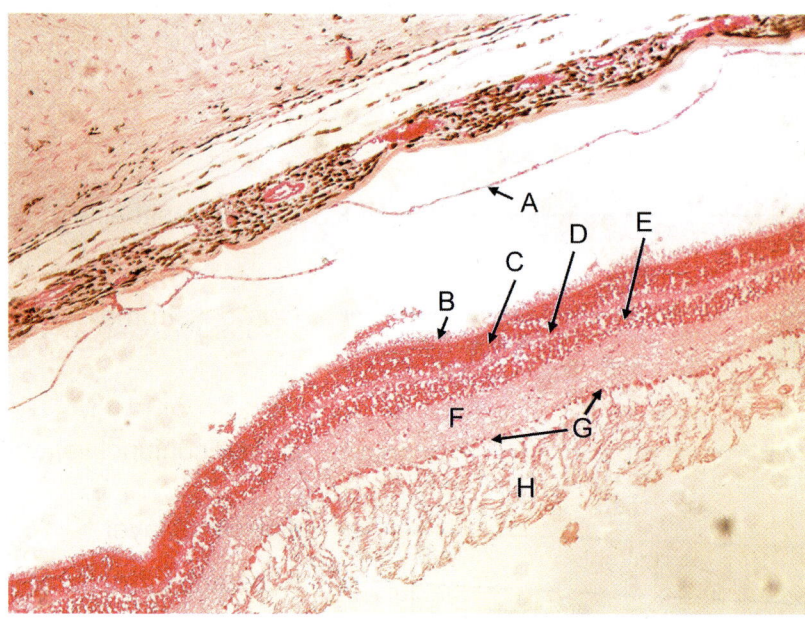

A	Pigment Cell Layer
B	Layer of Rod and Cones
C	Outer Nuclear Layer
D	Outer Plexiform Layer
E	Inner Nuclear Layer
F	Inner Plexiform Layer
G	Ganglion Cell Layer
H	Nerve Fiber Layer

Identification Points

1. **Ten-layered structure.**
2. **Outer most pigment cell layer, nuclear and ganglion cell layer are prominent.**
3. **Rods and cones present.**

Ten layers of retina are:
1. Pigment cell layer—outer most layer, cuboidal cells with melanin pigments.
   – Helps in absorption of light, prevent reflection. Phagocytose shed part of rods and cones.
2. Rod and cones—contains outer segments of photoreceptors (rods and cones).
3. External limiting membrane—formed by the processes of Muller's cells.
4. Outer nuclear layer—contains cell bodies of rods and cones. Rods associated with dim and black and white vision, cones with bright and color vision.
5. Outer plexiform layer—synapses between rods and cones with peripheral processes of bipolar cells.
6. Inner nuclear layer—cell bodies of bipolar cells, amacrine cells, horizontal cells.
7. Inner plexiform layer—synapses between central processes of bipolar with peripheral processes of ganglion cells.
8. Ganglion cell layer—large cell bodies of ganglion cells.
9. Nerve fiber layer—axons of ganglion cells which continue as optic nerve.
10. Inner limiting membrane—formed by the processes of Muller's cells.
    – Inner nine layers form neural layers of retina.
    – Rods and cones—photoreceptors.
    – Bipolar cells—first order neurons.
    – Ganglion cells—second order neurons.
    – Nutrition of retina:
      » Inner layers from central artery of retina.
      » Outer layers—diffusion from capillaries plexus of choroid.

72. RETINA

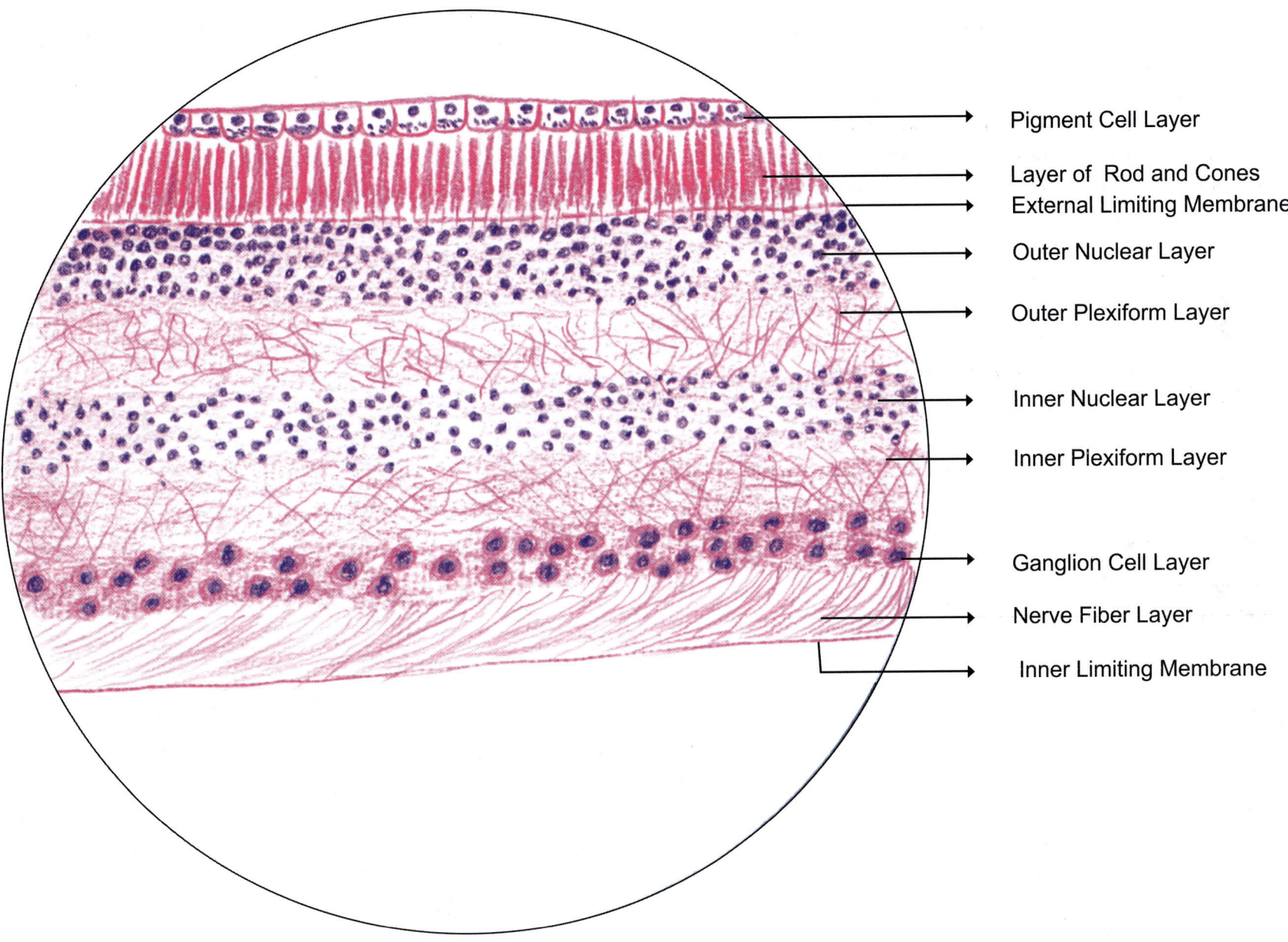

73. EYELID

EYELIDS

- It has the following layers from anterior to posterior.
- Skin—lined by stratified squamous keratinized epithelium.
  - Near the margin three to four rows of hairs are present forming the eyelashes.
  - Modified sweat glands called glands of Moll and sebaceous glands called glands of Zeis are associated with the eyelashes near the lid margin.
  - Beneath the skin, there is a layer of connective tissue which is devoid of fat.
- Muscle layer—made up of skeletal muscle (orbicularis oculi).
- Tarsal plate—forms the skeletal support for the lids.
  - Made up of dense connective tissue
  - Contains Meibomian glands which are sebaceous type of glands.
  - The ducts of these open on the lid margin.
  - The oily secretions from the glands coats over the lacrimal film and delays its evaporation.
- Conjunctiva—forms the innermost lining of the lid. It is made up of stratified columnar or cuboidal epithelium.

73. EYELID

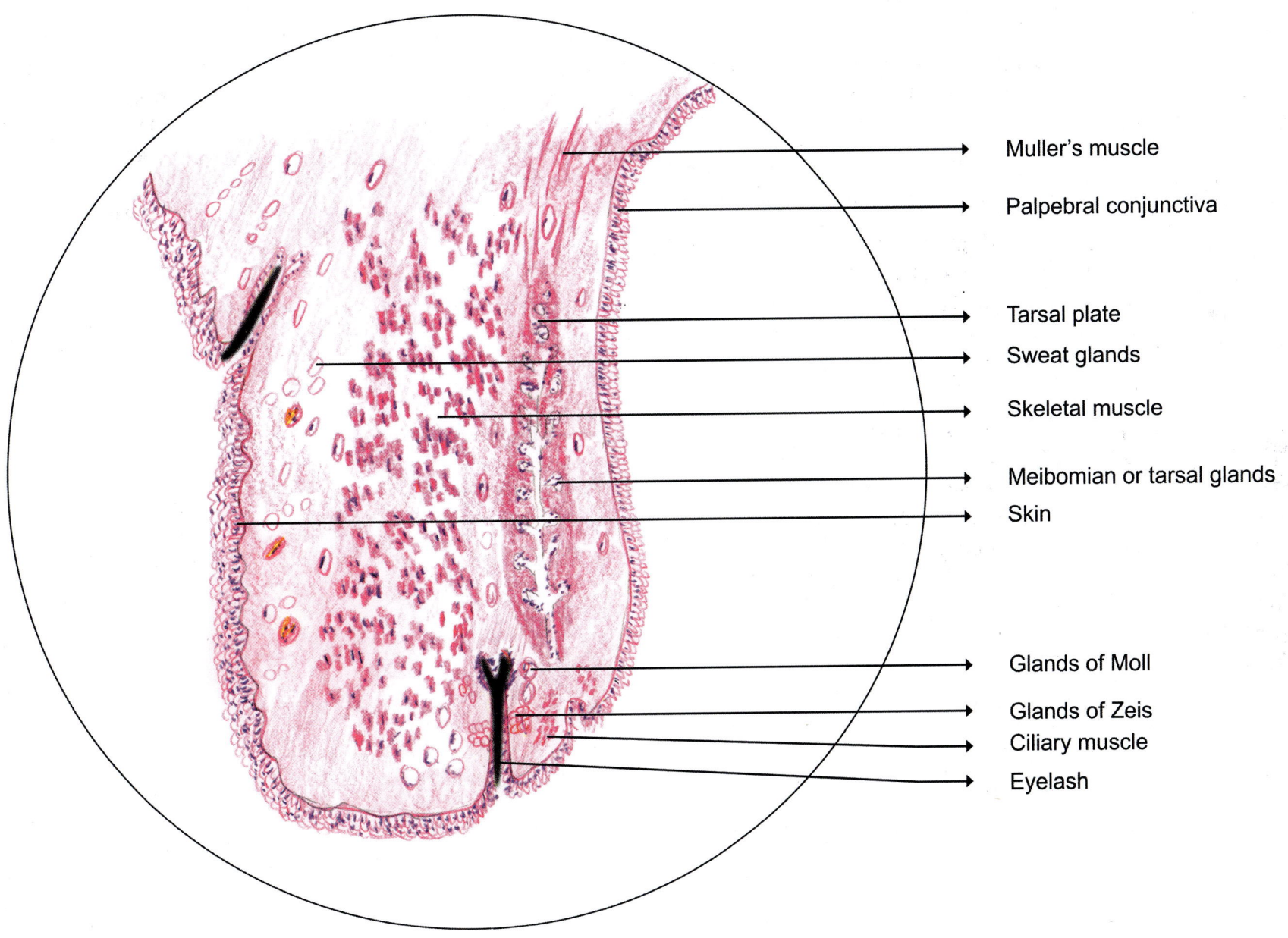

74. ORGAN OF CORTI

ORGAN OF CORTI

Inner ear is deep in the temporal bone, consists of communicating canals and cavities called bony labyrinth. Bony labyrinth is lined by membranous labyrinth. Bony labyrinth spirals around the central axis of spongy bone (modiolus) is called cochlea. Osseous spiral lamina projects from modiolus into the lumen of canal. Basilar membrane extends from spiral lamina to spiral ligament on the outer wall (thickening of periosteum and connective tissue). Vestibular membrane (Reissner's) membrane extends from spiral limbus to spiral ligament and separates scala media from scala vestibule.

Basilar membrane is a vascularized connective tissue membrane. Basilar membrane and vestibular membrane divides membranous labyrinth into 3 compartments—scala vestibuli, scala media and scala tympani. Scala media contains endolymph.

Organ of Corti—receptor organ of hearing:
- Consists outer three rows and inner single row of hair cells with supporting cells lying over the basilar membrane.
- Hair cells are receptors of hearing. Peripheral process of bipolar cells of spiral ganglion of cochlear nerve ends in the basal part of hair cells.
- Hair cells have stereocilia of different lengths and are embedded in tectorial membrane.
- Tectorial membrane extends from spiral limbus and covers the organ of Corti.

Supporting cells are:
- Pillar (rod) cells—have broad foot plates resting on basement membrane. Arranged as inner and outer row. Space enclosed between the two rows of pillar cells become tunnel of Corti and contains Corti lymph.
- Phalangeal cells (Dieters)—outer hair cells are supported by phalangeal cells resting on basilar membrane.
- Hensen's cells—lie lateral to the phalangeal cells. They support phalangeal cells and outer hair cells.
- Cells of Claudius—are lateral to Hensen's cells.
- Boettcher cells—lie on basilar membrane and are located deep to Claudius cells.

74. ORGAN OF CORTI

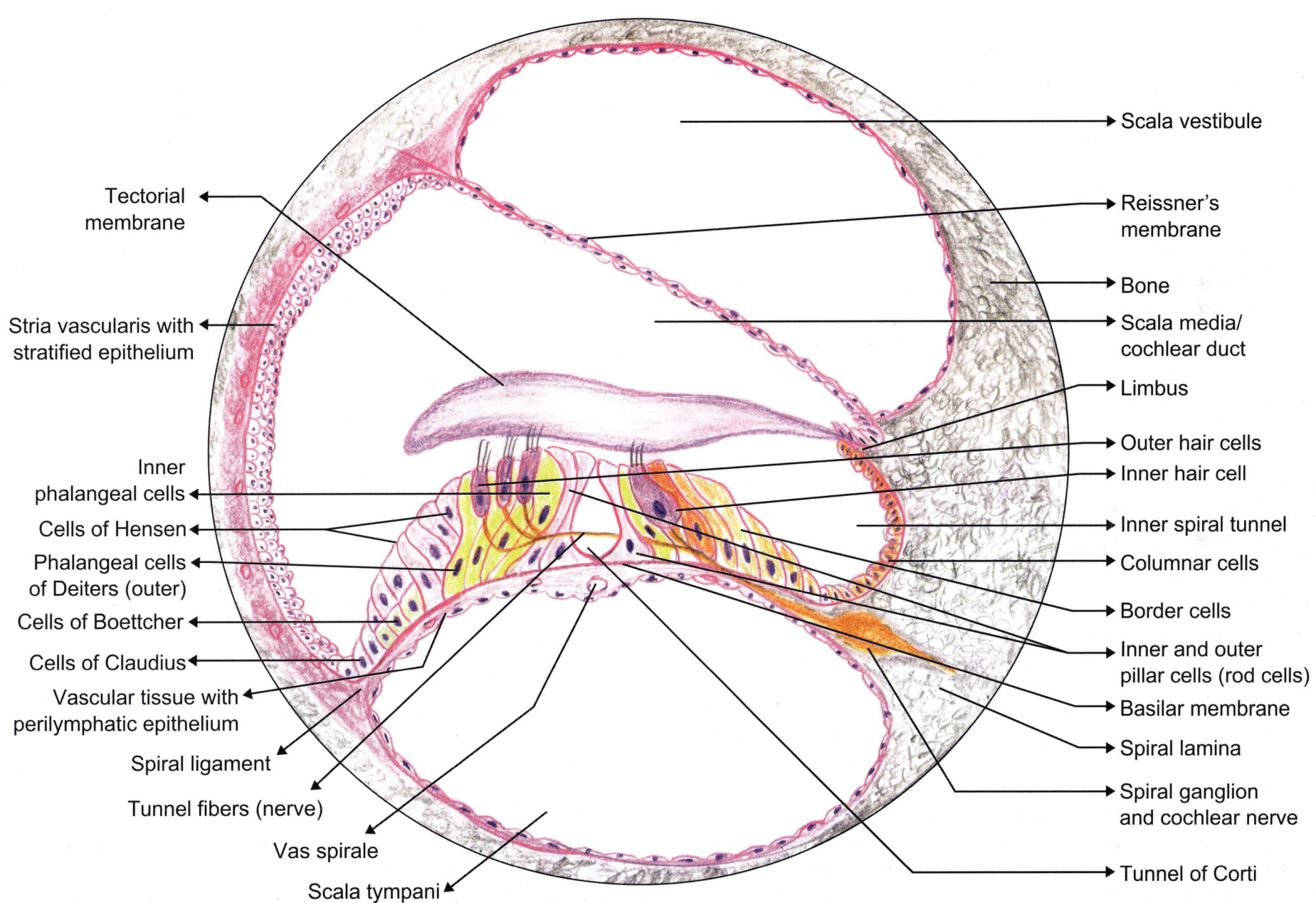

75. CEREBRUM

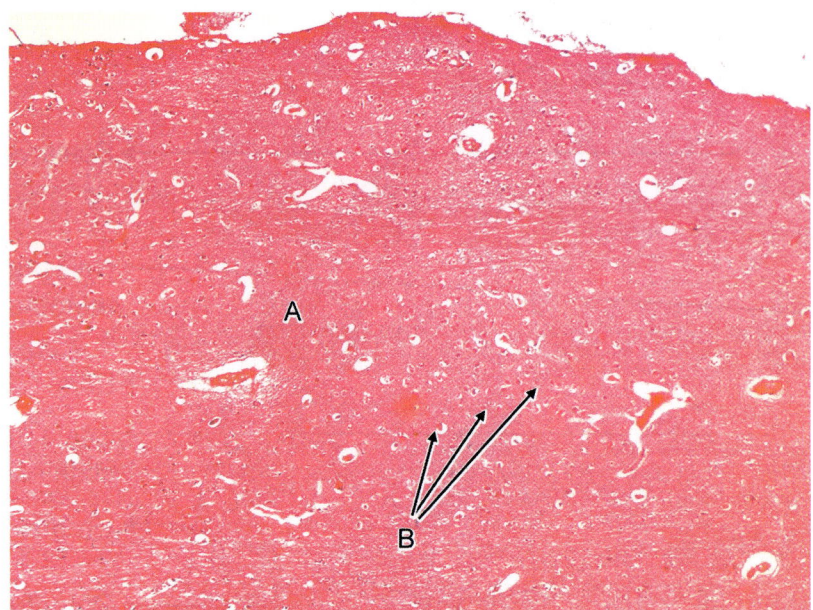

A	Cortex
B	Pyramidal Cells

Identification Points

Outer cortex—gray matter, inner medulla—white matter.
1. **Cortex—six-layered structure.**
2. **Main cell types—pyramidal and stellate cells.**
3. **Medulla contains myelinated nerve fibers.**

- Cerebral cortex described as six layered structure.
    1. Outer most layer is molecular or plexiform layer—mainly nerve fibers and few horizontal cells.
    2. External granular layer—contains predominantly stellate cells and few small pyramidal cells.
    3. External pyramidal layer—made up of small and medium-sized pyramidal cells with few stellate cells.
    4. Internal granular layer—made up of stellate cells and few pyramidal cells.
       There is a band of white fibers in the middle of this layer called external band of Baillarger.
    5. Internal pyramidal or ganglionic layer made up of large pyramidal cells of Betz. In this layer there is thin band of white fibers called internal band of Baillarger.
    6. Multiform or pleiomorphic layer with neurons of different sizes and shapes. Cells present are fusiform and cells of Martinotti.
- There is a considerable variation in structure from region to region. In motor cortex pyramidal cells predominate and in sensory cortex stellate cells are more in number.
- Pyramidal cells—pyramidal in shape with apex towards the surface of cortex. Axon arises from the base.

75. CEREBRUM

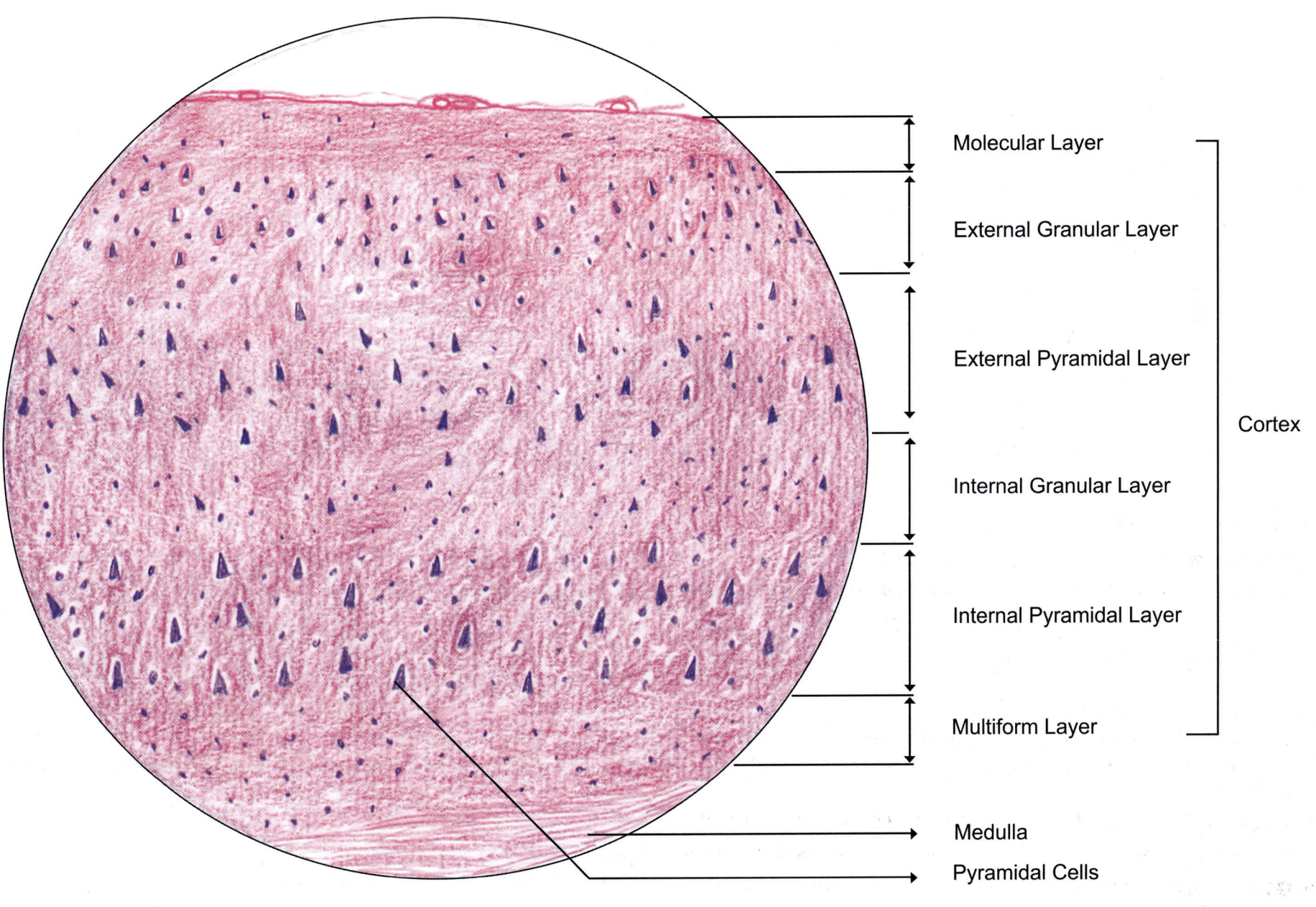

76. CEREBELLUM

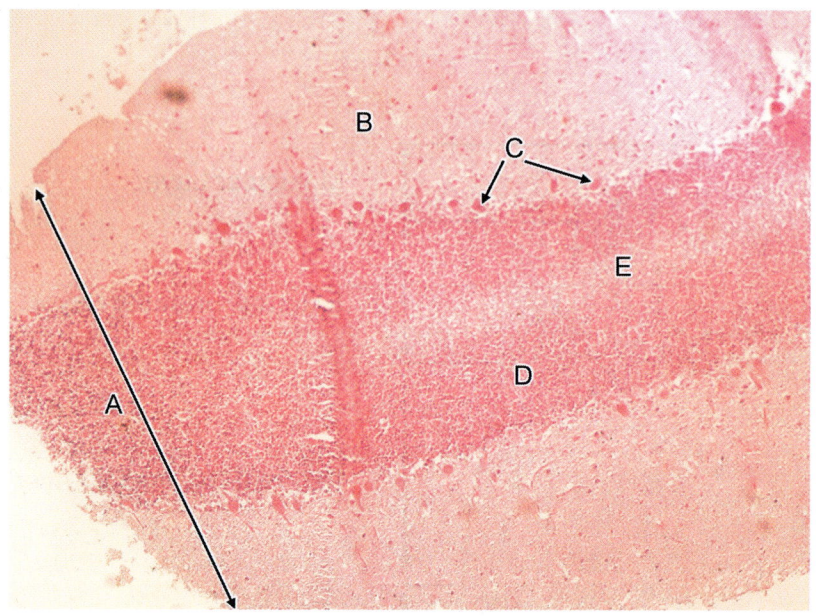

A	Folium
B	Molecular Layer
C	Purkinje Cell Layer
D	Granular Layer
E	White Matter

Identification Points

Cerebellar folia with outer cortex and inner medulla.

1. **Cortex—three-layered structure. Outer molecular, middle Purkinje cell and inner prominent granular cell layer seen.**
2. **Main cell types—Purkinje cells and granule cells.**
3. **Medulla is made up of white matter.**

Cortex—three-layered structure.
1. Outer molecular layer contains basket and stellate cells, dendrites of Purkinje cells and parallel fibers of granular cells.
2. Middle Purkinje cell—is single cell layer. These are large flask-shaped cells. Axons from the base of these cells enter medulla and synapse with cells of intracerebellar nuclei.
3. Inner granular cell layer made up of granule and Golgi cells and synaptic glomeruli.
   – Synaptic glomeruli formed by dendrites of granule cell, axon terminals of Golgi cell and terminal part of mossy fibers.
- Appearance of white matter is described as arbor vitae cerebelli. Made of myelinated nerve fibers.
- In cerebellar cortex only excitatory cell is granule cell. Remaining cells are inhibitory.
- Cerebellum is concerned with balance, co-ordination and muscle tone and posture.

76. CEREBELLUM

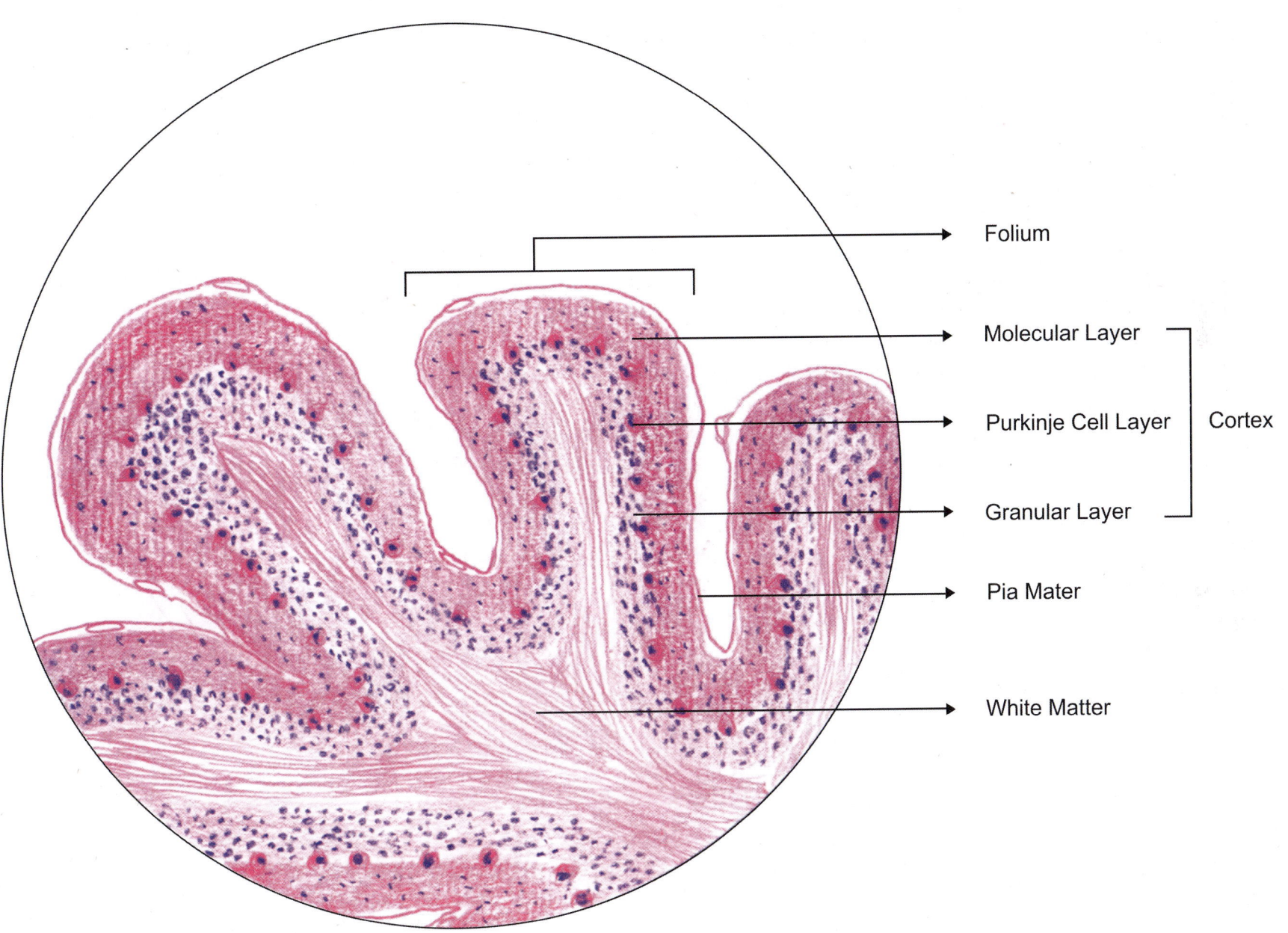

77. SPINAL CORD

Identification Points

1. **Central H-shaped gray matter with large anterior horns, narrow posterior horns.**
2. **Surrounding white matter with anterior deep median fissure.**

- Spinal cord extends from outer margin of foramen magnum to lower border of first lumbar vertebrae. It is part of central nervous system (CNS).
- It has three layers of meningeal coverings—dura mater, arachnoid, pia mater.
- Median anterior fissure is deep.
- Made up of central gray matter and outer white matter.
- Central H-shaped gray matter divided into anterior and posterior horns. Lateral horns are seen in thoracic segments.
- Anterior horns are larger than posterior. Contains multipolar motor neurons and interneurons.
- The gray matter of two sides is connected by gray commissure containing the central canal.
- White matter contains ascending and descending tracts. These are grouped as anterior, lateral and posterior columns.

77. SPINAL CORD

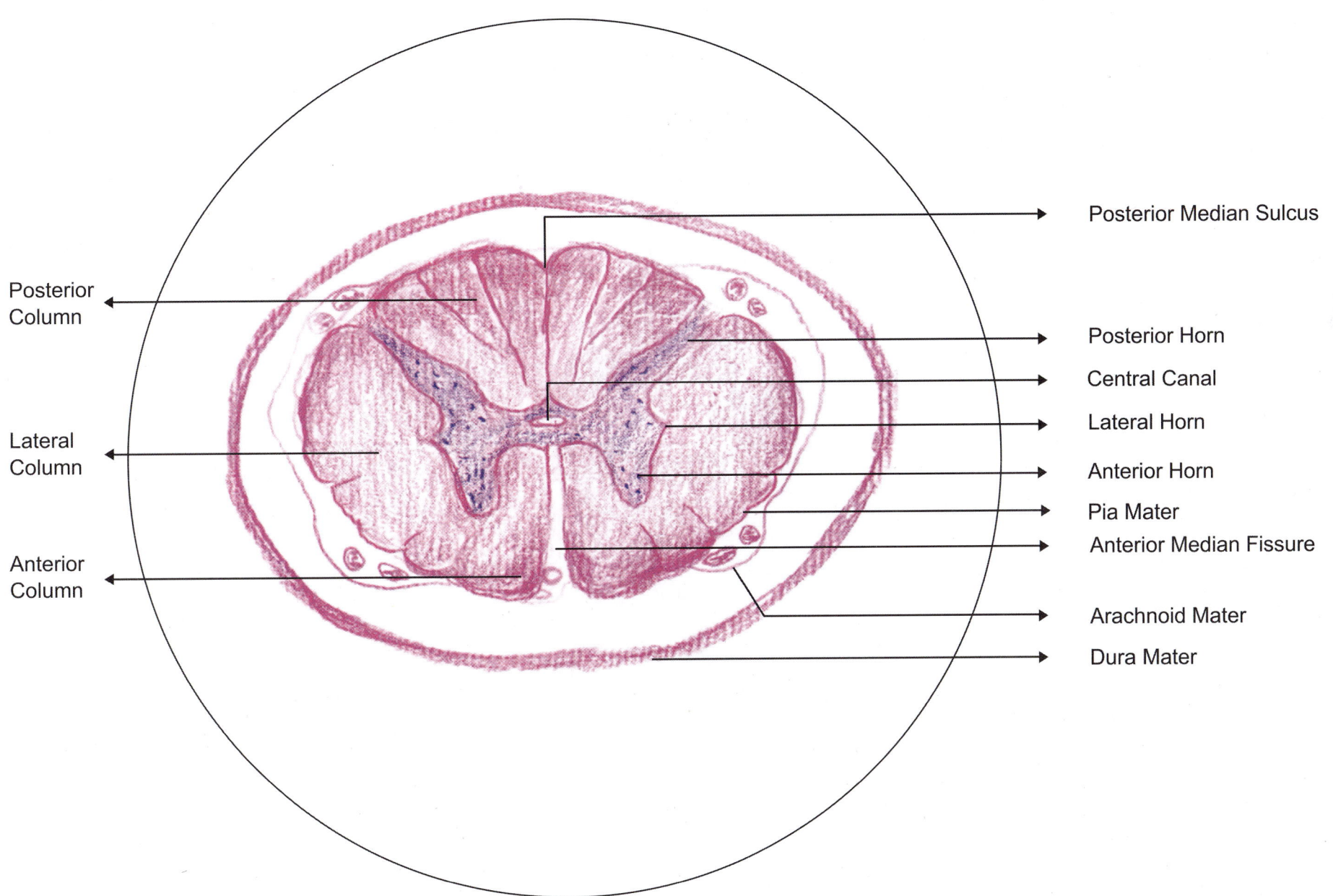

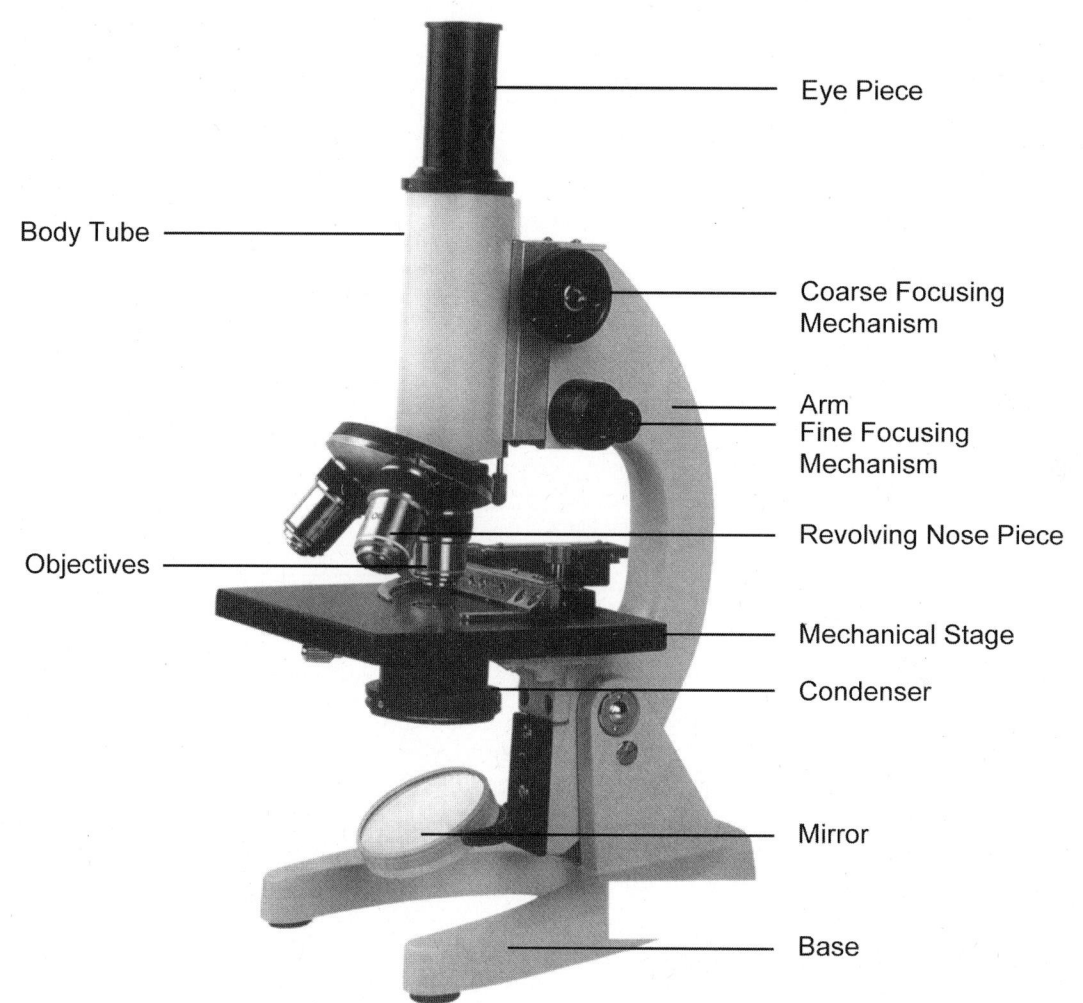